OTHER FAST FACTS BOOKS

Fast Facts for the WOUND CARE NURSE: Practical Wound Management in a Nutshell (*Kifer*)

Fast Facts About EKGs FOR NURSES: The Rules of Identifying EKGs in a Nutshell (*Landrum*)

Fast Facts for the CRITICAL CARE NURSE: Critical Care Nursing in a Nutshell (*Landrum*)

Fast Facts for the TRAVEL NURSE: Travel Nursing in a Nutshell (*Landrum*)

Fast Facts for the SCHOOL NURSE: School Nursing in a Nutshell, Second Edition (*Loschiavo*)

Fast Facts for MANAGING PATIENTS WITH A PSYCHIATRIC DISORDER: What RNs, NPs, and New Psych Nurses Need to Know (*Marshall*)

Fast Facts About SUBSTANCE USE DISORDERS: What Every Nurse, APRN, and PA Needs to Know (*Marshall, Spencer*)

Fast Facts About CURRICULUM DEVELOPMENT IN NURSING: How to Develop and Evaluate Educational Programs in a Nutshell, Second Edition (*McCoy, Anema*)

Fast Facts for the CATH LAB NURSE (*McCulloch*)

Fast Facts About NEUROCRITICAL CARE: A Quick Reference for the Advanced Practice Provider (*McLaughlin*)

Fast Facts for DEMENTIA CARE: What Nurses Need to Know in a Nutshell (*Miller*)

Fast Facts for HEALTH PROMOTION IN NURSING: Promoting Wellness in a Nutshell (*Miller*)

Fast Facts for STROKE CARE NURSING: An Expert Care Guide, Second Edition (*Morrison*)

Fast Facts for the MEDICAL OFFICE NURSE: What You Really Need to Know in a Nutshell (*Richmeier*)

Fast Facts for the PEDIATRIC NURSE: An Orientation Guide in a Nutshell (*Rupert, Young*)

Fast Facts About FORENSIC NURSING: What You Need to Know (*Scannell*)

Fast Facts About the GYNECOLOGICAL EXAM: A Professional Guide for NPs, PAs, and Midwives, Second Edition (*Secor, Fantasia*)

Fast Facts for the STUDENT NURSE: Nursing Student Success in a Nutshell (*Stabler-Haas*)

Fast Facts for CAREER SUCCESS IN NURSING: Making the Most of Mentoring in a Nutshell (*Vance*)

Fast Facts for the TRIAGE NURSE: An Orientation and Care Guide, Second Edition (*Visser, Montejano*)

Fast Facts for DEVELOPING A NURSING ACADEMIC PORTFOLIO: What You Really Need to Know in a Nutshell (*Wittmann-Price*)

Fast Facts for the HOSPICE NURSE: A Concise Guide to End-of-Life Care (*Wright*)

Fast Facts for the CLASSROOM NURSING INSTRUCTOR: Classroom Teaching in a Nutshell (*Yoder-Wise, Kowalski*)

Forthcoming FAST FACTS Books

Fast Facts About NEUROPATHIC PAIN: What Advanced Practice Nurses and Physician Assistants Need to Know (*Davies*)

Fact Facts in HEALTH INFORMATICS FOR NURSES (*Hardy*)

Fact Facts About NURSE ANESTHESIA (*Hickman*)

Fast Facts for the CARDIAC SURGERY NURSE, Third Edition (*Hodge*)

Fast Facts for the CRITICAL CARE NURSE: Critical Care Nursing, Second Edition (*Landrum*)

Fast Facts for the SCHOOL NURSE, Third Edition (*Loschiavo*)

Fast Facts on How to Conduct, Understand, and Maybe Even Love RESEARCH! For Nurses and Other Healthcare Providers (*Marshall*)

Fast Facts for DNP ROLE DEVELOPMENT: A Career Navigation Guide (*Menonna-Quinn, Genova*)

Visit www.springerpub.com to order.

FAST FACTS About
RELIGION FOR NURSES

Elizabeth Johnston Taylor, PhD, RN, FAAN, professor, Loma Linda University School of Nursing, Loma Linda, California, has pursued a program of research exploring the intersection of spirituality, religiosity, health, and nursing for 25 years. Her clinical experiences as an oncology nurse created for her a deep interest in these topics and led her to pursue a PhD (University of Pennsylvania), a postdoctoral fellowship (University of California, Los Angeles), clinical pastoral education, and training in spiritual direction.

The desire to help nurses understand and support patients' spiritual wellness during health-related transitions has motivated Dr. Johnston Taylor to write numerous articles and book chapters. Her books include *Spiritual Care: Nursing Theory, Research, and Practice* (2002), *What Do I Say? Talking With Patients About Spirituality* (2007), and *Religion: A Clinical Guide for Nurses* (Springer Publishing, 2012).

FAST FACTS About
RELIGION FOR NURSES

Implications for Patient Care

Elizabeth Johnston Taylor, PhD, RN, FAAN

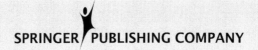
SPRINGER PUBLISHING COMPANY

Springer Publishing Company, LLC
11 West 42nd Street
New York, NY 10036
www.springerpub.com
http://connect.springerpub.com

Acquisitions Editor: Joe Morita
Compositor: Amnet Systems

ISBN: 978-0-8261-7826-8
e-book ISBN: 978-0-8261-7831-2
DOI: 10.1891/9780826178312

19 20 21 22 / 5 4 3 2 1

The author and the publisher of this Work have made every effort to use sources believed to be reliable to provide information that is accurate and compatible with the standards generally accepted at the time of publication. Because medical science is continually advancing, our knowledge base continues to expand. Therefore, as new information becomes available, changes in procedures become necessary. We recommend that the reader always consult current research and specific institutional policies before performing any clinical procedure. The author and publisher shall not be liable for any special, consequential, or exemplary damages resulting, in whole or in part, from the readers' use of, or reliance on, the information contained in this book. The publisher has no responsibility for the persistence or accuracy of URLs for external or third-party Internet websites referred to in this publication and does not guarantee that any content on such websites is, or will remain, accurate or appropriate.

Library of Congress Cataloging-in-Publication Data

Names: Johnston Taylor, Elizabeth, author.
Title: Fast facts about religion for nurses : implications for patient care /
  Elizabeth Johnston Taylor.
Description: New York, NY : Springer Publishing Company, LLC, 2019. | Series:
  Fast facts | Includes bibliographical references and index.
Identifiers: LCCN 2018061399 (print) | LCCN 2019000070 (ebook) | ISBN
  9780826178312 (ebook) | ISBN 9780826178268 (print : alk. paper)
Subjects: | MESH: Nursing Care | Religion | Culturally Competent Care |
  Nurse-Patient Relations
Classification: LCC RT41 (ebook) | LCC RT41 (print) | NLM WY 100.1 | DDC
  610.73—dc23
LC record available at https://lccn.loc.gov/2018061399

Contact us to receive discount rates on bulk purchases.
We can also customize our books to meet your needs.
For more information please contact sales@springerpub.com

Elizabeth Johnston Taylor: https://orcid.org/0000-0002-6790-8801

*Given the nature of their work with people encountering
health challenges and adversities, nurses frequently provide witness for
the religious struggles and stirrings of those for whom they provide care.
Indeed, the caring nurse often becomes the hands and face—or
embodiment—of Divine Love (i.e., God, Allah, Great Mystery, Jesus,
Brahman, Ahura Mazda, or whatever name and characterization reflects
human understanding about the source of love).
Thus, this book is dedicated to every compassionate nurse.*

Contents

Contents

Preface

"Humans are religious by nature," wrote religion scholar Nadeau (2014). "They seek patterns of meaning and action that are ultimately transformative. As such, religion is a model of and a model for reality, as experienced, by individuals in the context of social, natural, and cosmic existence" (p. 8). Or as my seriously ill friend, Kandace, put it, "Religion is what people use to understand mystery." Another simple definition for religion is what Elizabeth Duke offered at a 2018 New Zealand Quaker meeting: It is "doing spirituality together." Regardless of the scope and emphasis a definition of religion offers, religion is a salient and integral aspect of human culture.

Given the importance of religion for humans and its function to provide them with transformative meaning and guide action, it is particularly important for them when they get sick, become disabled, celebrate a new life, mourn a loss, or face death. And it is at just such times as these that nurses typically meet a person, family, group, or community. Thus, although it is unrealistic to expect nurses to become experts in comparative religions, they ought to have a minimal awareness of diverse religions to be able to ask a patient pertinent questions and plan religiously sensitive care—thus, this book.

Often in nursing texts, information about religions is either incorrect or essentialized. It typically fails to provide understanding for why one may perform certain rituals or hold certain beliefs. It also usually fails to recognize the variety of religious perspectives that exist even within a religious tradition. Thus, I have attempted to write this book so that it allows a busy nurse to not only quickly access information but also get the information with some context. Yes, this is a glorified cookbook. For more depth, the reader is referred to *Religion: A Clinical Guide for Nurses*.

What religions are included? What information for each religion is included? Religions included are those most likely to be encountered by a Western, English-speaking, first world nurse—the nurse who can obtain this book. However, several religions with smaller numbers of adherents (yet more than 200,000 or so in North America) were included if their religion involved significant health-related implications. An attempt was made to delimit the information about each religion to only that which would provide necessary context or entail practice implications relevant for a nurse. For example, details about funerary customs and decision making about using genetic therapeutics were generally not included, as these would be the domain of a mortician or genetics counselor. It should also be noted that for many religions, there are no explicit directives to guide healthcare decision making; therefore, the information provided is sometimes skimpy.

Bibliography

Duke, E. (2018). Can religion speak truth? *Dunedin (New Zealand) Friends' Epistle.* Retrieved from http://fwcc.world/wp-content/uploads/2018/06/Aotearoa-New-Zealand-YM-2018.pdf

Nadeau, R. L. (2014). *Asian religions: A cultural perspective.* West Sussex, UK: Wiley Blackwell.

Taylor, E. J. (Ed.). (2012). *Religion: A clinical guide for nurses.* New York, NY: Springer Publishing.

Acknowledgments

No book is written without help. My deep gratitude is extended to my ever-faithful personal and professional enabler, husband Lyndon Johnston Taylor; my incredibly encouraging and open-minded editors at Springer, Margaret Zuccarini (publisher emerita), Joe Morita (senior editor), Rachel Landes (associate editor), and Hannah Hicks (assistant editor); Dr. Sharon Hinton at the Westberg Institute for Faith Community Nursing who mobilized numerous reviewers for me; and the following expert reviewers who carefully examined and edited their respective book chapter(s) so that the contents would be accurate and positive. Sometimes their input was substantial, and I was inspired by their willingness to teach all of us.

Chapter 2:   Cynthia Duncan, PhD (Eñi Acho)

Chapter 3:   Randolph Dobbs

Chapter 4:   Reverend Jundo Gregory Gibbs

Chapter 5:   Eva Meyers, PhD, RN; Janet Meyers, BS, RN

Chapter 6:   Jacqueline Mickley, PhD, RN

Chapter 7:   Linda Garner, RN; Helen Wordsworth, RGN

Chapter 8:   Vickie Franklin, RN

Chapter 10: Blaine A. Winters, DNP, ACNP-BC

Chapter 11: Carol Gaskamp, PhD, RN; Reverend Greg Gaskamp

Chapter 12: Susie Enfield, MSN, RN; Teresa Darnall, DM, MSN, RN, CNE

Chapter 13: Marsha Stevens-Pino, RN

Chapter 14: Amy Armanious, DNP, MSN, MSOL, RN

Chapter 15: Marion Harris, MSN, RN, PHN; Bishop Jerry Wayne Macklin

Chapter 16: M. Jerdone Davis, EdD, MACE, RN

Chapter 17: Ruth Fiedler, EdD, RN, APRN-BC, CNE; Laurie Rippe, RN

Chapter 18: Martha E. F. Highfield, PhD, RN; Ronald Highfield, PhD

Chapter 19: Dorothy Mayernik, RN; Deborah Meiklejohn, RN; Mary Ann Serra, RN; Linda Walsh, BSN, RN, FCN; Lynne M. Hutchison, DNP, FNP-BC; Reverend Mr. Thomas K. Badger

Chapter 20: Marietta Kellum, RN

Chapter 21: Most reviewers for other Christian chapters also reviewed this chapter.

Chapter 22: Lisa Roberts, DrPH, MSN, RN, FNP-BC, CHES, FAANP; Roger E. Hedlund, PhD

Chapter 23: Rabbi Wynne R. Waugaman, PhD, CRNA, FAAN

Chapter 24: Rabbi Wynne R. Waugaman, PhD, CRNA, FAAN

Chapter 25: Rabbi Wynne R. Waugaman, PhD, CRNA, FAAN

Chapter 26: Nancy Romanchek, RN

Chapter 29: Robin PetersonLund (Tasunka Wakan Nagi Win [*Sacred Horse Spirit Woman*], of Oglala Lakota, Wazizi band, Pine Ridge), PhD, RN, CNS, FNP-BC; Mary Isaacson, PhD, RN, CHPN

Chapter 30: Savitri Singh-Carlson, PhD, APHN-BC, FAAN

Chapter 31: John Jones, PhD

Chapter 32: Artemis Javanshir, Mandana Pishdadi, Maneck Bhujwala, Lovji Cama

Supporting Patient Religiosity: The Five Ws

Introduction

Any news story begins by answering the five *W* questions of *who*, *what*, *where*, *when*, and *why*. Thus, we begin by addressing these questions as they relate to nurses providing patients with religiously sensitive care. The *how* question is often also included in a news story. Given that this question of how to care for the religious patient is the prompt for this book, it is addressed in all the subsequent chapters (see Box 1.1, however, for some guiding principles).

BOX 1.1   GUIDING PRINCIPLES FOR ADDRESSING RELIGIOSITY

- Remember that every religious person will interpret religious beliefs and implement religious practices in his or her unique way. Avoid making assumptions; instead, assess.
- Be at ease with not knowing everything about every religion. Let your desire to provide care in a religio-culturally competent manner prompt inquiry and sensitivity.
- Be nonjudgmental. While this does not mean you need to agree with the patient, it also means you ought not to debate theology. When you have the urge to convince a patient of a "better" way to believe (i.e., your way), remember that it may actually be your own theological insecurity driving this desire.

(continued)

BOX 1.1   GUIDING PRINCIPLES FOR ADDRESSING RELIGIOSITY (*continued*)

- Behave respectfully. This does not mean you feel respectful (but it does help!).
- Avoid framing faith-related concerns as problems to fix. Instead, remember they are a salient aspect of culture and express one's view of the world and how to live.

What?

Over the past few decades, nurses have increasingly embraced the concept of spirituality and avoided discussions of religion. This distinction of spirituality from religion reflects a societal trend yet fails to recognize that spirituality originally was conceived of as the personal, subjective aspect of religious experience (Steinhauser et al., 2017). Koenig (2011), a physician scholar in the area of religion and health, offered a definition of religion that reflects contemporary thinking: "An organized system of beliefs, practices, and symbols designed to facilitate closeness to the transcendent or the Divine and foster an understanding of one's relationship and responsibilities with others living in community" (p. 197). Like other definitions, this emphasizes not only the beliefs and practices but also the relational or corporate aspect of religion.

Over the past several decades, social scientists have proposed that religion is composed of multiple dimensions. Pearce, Hayward, and Pearlman (2017) empirically tested if and how five dimensions of religiosity identified in this body of theorizing existed; from statistical analyses of very large national samples of adolescents, they established that these dimensions existed and were interrelated. Thus, the following dimensions of religiosity are apropos for U.S. adults and adolescents:

- Religious beliefs (the ideology or set of beliefs one has about the supernatural, afterlife, meaning of life and suffering, and so forth)
- Religious exclusivity (the orthodoxy, dogmatism, fundamentalism, or beliefs about absolutes—rules about what is right and wrong)
- External practice (the social involvement or group membership in a faith community)
- Personal practice (the personal dedication and devotionalism)
- Religious salience (the importance of religion in the hierarchy of a person's life; Pearce et al., 2017)

These categories begin to describe the complexity of religion; thus, they provide nurses with a lens through which to understand patients' religiosity.

Why?

Several reasons support why nurses must provide care that is sensitive to patient religiosity:

- Religion is global, prevalent, and salient in the lives of humans. In 2017, the world's religions were distributed as follows:
  - Christianity: 31.2%
  - Islam: 24.1%
  - Hinduism: 15.1%
  - Buddhism: 6.9%
  - Folk religions: 5.7%
  - Other religions: 0.8%
  - Judaism: 0.2%

  Only 16% of the world population was unaffiliated (e.g., atheist, agnostic; Pew Research Center, 2017).
- Ethical and professional mandates underscore that nursing care be respectful of patients' creed and culture and that it be holistic—including care for the spiritual dimension of persons (American Nurses Association, 2015; International Council of Nurses, 2012).
- Evidence from over 3,300 studies documents that religiosity and spirituality are associated with or contribute to health outcomes significantly and positively (Koenig, King, & Carson, 2012). (About 80% of these studies examined religiosity or spirituality in relation to psychological factors.) Frequency of religious practices (e.g., attending religious services or prayer) and positive religious beliefs (e.g., "God loves me") are associated with indicators of physical and psychological health. More specifically:
  - Religious beliefs affect how one interprets illness, tragedy, and suffering. Furthermore, negative religious beliefs or interpretations that cause an inner religious struggle are associated with depression, anxiety, and other poor outcomes (e.g., Fitchett, Winter-Pfandler, & Pargament, 2014). For example, findings from a well-designed study of 101 Americans with end-stage congestive heart failure found that religious or spiritual struggle predicted future hospitalization and physical functioning (Park, Wortmann, & Edmondson, 2011).
  - Religious beliefs also influence how one pursues health and makes healthcare decisions (Taylor, in press). For example, the belief that God can work a miracle may contribute to a decision

to reject chemotherapy or not sign a do-not-resuscitate (DNR) order. Religious beliefs about modesty and hygiene, of course, will have an impact on healthcare preferences, too.

- Some religious beliefs and practices can have immediate implications for physical health (e.g., what foods or drink to ingest, certain ascetic practices such as pilgrimages and fasting).
- Religious—and even nonreligious—patients use religious practices to cope with health challenges and to promote overall well-being (e.g., Morton, Lee, & Martin, 2017; VanderWeele et al., 2017). Common practices include meditation, yoga, and prayer, which originate from ancient religions.
- When healthcare professionals support patient religiosity and/or spirituality, this support is associated with patient satisfaction and other desirable outcomes (Taylor, in press). Indeed, in one study of over 600 Asian patients, nurse-provided spiritual care was the most important mediator explaining the relationship between met spiritual needs and patient satisfaction (Hodge, Sun, & Wolosin, 2014). Although this literature fails to describe the nature of nurse-provided "spiritual care," it is likely that it often entailed supporting religious needs, as that is what nurses and patients often consider spiritual care to be.

Thus, if nursing care is to be ethical and respectful, informed by evidence that demonstrates low religious struggle and high spiritual or religious well-being are associated with health, and cognizant of the reality that religious beliefs and practices affect health and healthcare, then nurses can only conclude that religiously sensitive care is imperative. Arguably, nurses are careless if they fail to provide religiously sensitive care for those who are religious or experiencing religious struggle.

Who?

The religiosity of the care recipient is associated with how welcomed religious support from a nurse is; that is, more religious patients and family caregivers do want care that is religiously sensitive (Taylor, 2006; Taylor & Brander, 2013). Those who are more likely to be religious include:

- Those of African (especially) or Latino descent
- Women
- Persons who are over 50 years old
- Those who are married
- Those who have not attended college (Brown, Taylor, & Chatters, 2015; Pew Research Center, 2018)

It is always possible, however, that a minimally religious person (or even someone who has rejected religion), when facing a significant health challenge or threat to life, may seek to intensify his or her religious experience or struggle to address religious doubts, questions, or regrets (e.g., Exline, Park, Smyth, & Carey, 2011). Thus, as Fitchett, Murphy, and King (2017, p. 101) advocated with their spiritual screening protocol, if a patient identifies that "there ever was a time when religion/spirituality was important," then attention ought to be paid.

Where?

In the United States, persons living in certain regions are also more likely to be religious. Per capita, the central states (from North Dakota and Minnesota to Texas) and the South (or "Bible Belt") are more religious than those in the West (except Utah, densely populated by Latter-day Saints) and northern New England (Association of Religion Data Archives, 2010). Globally, however, except in the Asia-Pacific continents where 75% of persons are unaffiliated with a religion, high percentages of citizens are affiliated with a religion (88% in Europe, 94% or more in remaining continents; Pew Research Center, 2017). These data indicate that regardless of where you practice nursing, more often than not, a patient will have some religious affiliation.

When?

Given that ethical and empirical prompts direct nurses to maintain a stance of respect for all patients' creeds and cultures, religiously sensitive care should always be provided. Some circumstances, however, particularly merit attention to the religious beliefs and practices of patients. These include times when the patient is:

- Unable to independently participate in religious rituals and requires assistance to do so
- Facing a major decision about healthcare that may be shaped by religious beliefs
- Struggling with difficult emotions such as depression or anger, which may be because of unhelpful religious beliefs or may find resolution from helpful religious beliefs or practices
- Confronting a serious illness, disability, or death—which often shatters one's worldview

Thus, inquiring about health-related religious beliefs and practices at admission or at times listed here can assist the nurse to know how to provide religiously sensitive care. Table 1.1 provides a list of assessment questions.

Table 1.1

Questions and Tips for Assessing Patient Religiosity	
Question	**Comments**
How important is your religion/faith to you now? (If not important, ask if it ever was before.)	Responses could be obtained in a variety of ways: a visual analog scale, verbally "on a scale of 0–10," or left open.
	If patient indicates there has been a change in importance of faith, this may indicate a religious struggle.
	This dimension of religiosity is highly correlated with other dimensions (Pearce et al., 2017), thus being a good indicator of overall religiosity.
I noticed (religious object or reference [e.g., religious jewelry, artwork, music, statement made by patient]); it'd be helpful for me to know more about how your faith affects you now.	This type of question can be used generically, outside of a formal assessment context. Only ask about manifestations of patient religiosity, however, if it is for therapeutic or health-related purposes (vs. curiosity or desire to evangelize).
Which of your cultural, spiritual, or religious beliefs and practices would be important for our healthcare team to know about? Are there any beliefs or practices that you especially need us to support?	Including the term *cultural* may make the question more comfortable and applicable.
	Note what language the patient uses (e.g., faith, values, worldview); use that language when possible.
	Avoid wording questions that place the patient in a passive position; rather frame the questions to indicate a desire to collaborate.
For many people, religious or spiritual beliefs influence the way they cope with illness (or disability or death or "times like this"). How is it for you?	Note the neutral wording of *influence*, instead of the biased language of *help* or *harm*.
	Patients prefer questions that frame spiritual resources in a positive way.
	Note the introductory sentence. Given the sensitive nature of the topic, such an introductory statement may be helpful for any querying about religion.

Final Considerations

A few final observations are essential to consider.

Not All Adventists (or Zoroastrians) Are Alike

As the multiple dimensions of religiosity listed previously imply, religiosity is highly variable even when it is not visible. To illustrate, the

Pew Research Center (2018) surveyed Americans and asked, "Do you believe in God or not?" Although 90% ultimately reported that they did believe in God, only 56% believed in "God as described in the Bible," while the remainder believed in some "higher power/spiritual force"—labeled by 23% as "God" and not by 9%. Even belief in God means different things to different people.

Furthermore, within religious traditions or denominations, differences in doctrinal interpretation and religious practices will exist. (One Jew may believe in heaven, while another does not. One Seventh-Day Adventist may play sports on Sabbath [Saturday], while another does not.) Likewise, within a family that shares the same religious affiliation, there can be such variations. Indeed, within an individual's life span, religious faith develops—or stagnates. Thus, to read about a religion in this book and assume that this information will completely apply to any patient who is an adherent to that religion is fallacious. Nurses must adapt the content of the forthcoming chapters to provide patient-specific care.

Religion Can Be Harmful

Although the thousands of studies investigating religion or spirituality in relation to health quite consistently indicate religiosity and health are positively linked (Koenig et al., 2012), a caveat must be noted. Some religious practices and beliefs can be harmful. For example, refusal of a vaccination or Western medical treatment for religious reasons could cause disease or death. For the person of faith, however, to disobey God or counter beliefs would be a greater harm. Thus, for the nurse wanting to respect the religion of a patient whose beliefs are considered harmful, it is important to (a) clarify these beliefs (possibly engaging the patient's religious leader in this process); (b) offer the nursing perspective and boundaries about helpful care; and (c) negotiate what care to provide.

Positive religious coping, manifested in a secure attachment to a benevolent God and connectedness with a faith community, is associated with adaptation (Pargament & Ano, 2006). In contrast, negative religious coping is maladaptive. It can involve a sense of abandonment and punishment by God, doubts about the power of God, thinking that one's illness is caused by a dark or devilish force, and isolation from one's religious community. A significant minority (or in some studies, over 50%) of patients use negative religious coping (Taylor, in press). When there is evidence of negative religious coping, it is important that the nurses seek consultation from a spiritual care expert so that this harmful religious thinking can be addressed therapeutically.

Nurses Can Be Harmful

Religion is an intimate and intricate, personal and private topic for many patients. Indeed, for some it may be a taboo topic. Hence, utmost sensitivity is required from the nurse. Ethical nursing care directs that nurses address patient religious needs only if doing so is for health reasons (e.g., to increase comfort, introduce coping strategies, support decision making, or assist patients to worship as they desire). The nurse must avoid any appearance of coercion and provide care that reflects patient preferences (Taylor, in press). Ethical religiously sensitive nursing care, however, can improve nurse and patient outcomes.

Bibliography

American Nurses Association. (2015). *The code of ethics for nurses with interpretive statements*. Silver Spring, MD: Author.

Association of Religion Data Archives. (2010). *U.S. congregational membership: Maps*. Retrieved from http://www.thearda.com/mapsReports/maps/Ardamap.asp?GRP=1&map1=3

Brown, R. K., Taylor, R. J., & Chatters, L. M. (2015). Race/ethnic and social-demographic correlates of religious non-involvement in America: Findings from three national surveys. *Journal of Black Studies, 46*(4), 335–362. doi:10.1177/0021934715573168

Exline, J. J., Park, C. L., Smyth, J. M., & Carey, M. P. (2011). Anger toward God: Social-cognitive predictors, prevalence, and links with adjustment to bereavement and cancer. *Journal of Personality and Social Psychology, 100*(1), 129–148. doi:10.1037/a0021716

Fitchett, G., Murphy, P., & King, S. D. W. (2017). Examining the validity of the Rush Protocol to screen for religious/spiritual struggle. *Journal of Health Care Chaplaincy, 23*(3), 98–112. doi:10.1080/08854726.2017.1294861

Fitchett, G., Winter-Pfändler, U., & Pargament, K. I. (2014). Struggle with the divine in Swiss patients visited by chaplains: Prevalence and correlates. *Journal of Health Psychology, 19*(8), 966–976. doi:10.1177/1359105313482167

Hodge, D. R., Sun, F., & Wolosin, R. J. (2014). Hospitalized Asian patients and their spiritual needs: Developing a model of spiritual care. *Journal of Aging & Health, 26*(3), 380–400. doi:10.1177/0898264313516995

International Council of Nurses. (2012). *The ICN code of ethics for nurses*. Geneva, Switzerland: Author.

Koenig, H. G. (2011). *Spirituality & health research: Methods, measurement, statistics, and resource*. West Conshohocken, PA: Templeton.

Koenig, H. G., King, D., & Carson, V. B. (2012). *Handbook of religion and health* (2nd ed.). New York: Oxford University Press.

Morton, K. R., Lee, J. W., & Martin, L. R. (2017). Pathways from religion to health: Mediation by psychosocial and lifestyle mechanisms. *Psychology of Religion & Spirituality, 9*(1), 106–117. doi:10.1037/rel0000091

Pargament, K. I., & Ano, G. G. (2006). Spiritual resources and struggles in coping with medical illness. *Southern Medical Journal, 99*(10), 1161–1162. doi:10.1097/01.smj.0000242847.40214.b6

Park, C. L., Wortmann, J. H., & Edmondson, D. (2011). Religious struggle as a predictor of subsequent mental and physical well-being in advanced heart failure patients. *Journal of Behavioral Medicine, 34*(6), 426–436. doi:10.1007/s10865-011-9315-y

Pearce, L. D., Hayward, G. M., & Pearlman, J. A. (2017). Measuring five dimensions of religiosity across adolescence. *Review of Religious Research, 59,* 367–393. doi:10.1007/s13644-017-0291-8

Pew Research Center. (2017). *The changing global religious landscape.* Retrieved from http://www.pewforum.org/2017/04/05/the-changing-global-religious-landscape

Pew Research Center. (2018). *When Americans say they believe in God, what do they mean?* Retrieved from http://www.pewforum.org/2018/04/25/when-americans-say-they-believe-in-god-what-do-they-mean

Steinhauser, K., Fitchett, G., Handzo, G., Johnson, K., Koenig, H., Pargament, K., . . . Balboni, T. (2017). State of the science of spirituality and palliative care research part I: Definitions, measurement, and outcomes. *Journal of Pain and Symptom Management, 54*(3), 428–440. doi:10.1016/j.jpainsymman.2017.07.028

Taylor, E. J. (in press). Health outcomes of religious and spiritual belief, behavior, and belonging: Implications for healthcare professionals. In F. Timmons & S. Caldeira (Eds.), *Spirituality in healthcare: Quality and performance.* Paris, France: Springer Nature.

Taylor, E. J., & Brander, P. (2013). Hospice patient and family carer perspectives on nurse spiritual assessment. *Journal of Hospice & Palliative Nursing, 15*(6), 347–354. doi:10.1097/NJH.0b013e3182979695

Taylor, E. J. (2006). Prevalence and associated factors of spiritual needs among patients with cancer and family caregivers. *Oncology Nursing Forum, 33*(4), 729–735. doi:10.1188/06.ONF.729-735

VanderWeele, T. J., Yu, J., Cozier, Y. C., Wise, L., Argentieri, M. A., Rosenberg, L., . . . Shields, A. E. (2017). Attendance at religious services, prayer, religious coping, and religious/spiritual identity as predictors of all-cause mortality in the Black Women's Health Study. *American Journal of Epidemiology, 185*(7), 515–522. doi:10.1093/aje/kww179

2

Afro-Caribbean and Traditional Yoruba Religions

Religions most like **Lucumí** (the most prevalent Afro-Caribbean religion in the United States) will be the focus of this chapter. Because the smaller Jamaican religions (e.g., Obeah, Revivalism) are substantially different from the other Afro-Caribbean religions, they are omitted. **Rastafarianism**, however, is briefly discussed because of its unique health-related prescriptions.

Other Names and Similar Religious Traditions

Various religions prevalent in the Caribbean include **Candomblé** (from Brazil); **Lucumí** (also known as **Santería** and **Regla de Ocha**, **"the Way of the Orichás"**) and **Palo Mayombe**—also known as **Las Reglas de Congo** (from Cuba); and **Vodoun** or **Voodoo** (from Haiti). **Yoruba**, a traditional African religion increasingly practiced among African Americans in North America, is similar. Within these traditions, other denominations or subgroups with separate names may exist.

Social and Historical Background

These Afro-Caribbean religions result from the interplay of indigenous religions, spiritism (beliefs originating in Europe about how the living can communicate with the dead), the African religions of the slaves brought to the region, and the religions of the Caribbean colonizers (mostly Catholicism). Although there is substantial diversity within and between these religions, the following characteristics are often shared. First, while there may or may not be a creator god, there is a pantheon of semidivine entities (deities) and the spirits of ancestors who are venerated. These deities and spirits assist to guide humans and nature. Second, these deities are invoked through prayers and divinations to intervene on behalf of those seeking help. The rituals are led by a priest or priestess usually in the presence of practitioners. Third, often these rituals are observed in secret. This is because the process of initiation provides instruction for practitioners that is unnecessary for "outsiders" to know. The secrecy may also reflect the centuries of persecution experienced by practitioners while under the political control of the colonizing Christians. Fourth, generally, these religions are not officially organized, and leadership is typically passed down through family lineage. Fifth, whereas some devotees may be initiated (via a process that could be one or several years long), some may not be, and they seek out a priest or priestess only when in need. Sixth, given the theological flexibility of Afro-Caribbean religions, when colonizers imposed their religion (typically Catholicism), the indigenous people responded by becoming more pluralistic. For example, enforced Catholic holy days became opportunities for Afro-Caribbean religious holidays; today, many similarities can be observed between deities and saints. Both Afro-Caribbean and Catholic religiosity often concurrently permeates practitioners' lives. Ultimately, these religions offer practitioners beliefs about the importance of living a moral life and living in harmony with others and with nature; such living brings blessings from God and the spirits. Thus:

- Puerto Rican, Jamaican, Trinidadian, Cuban, and other patients with strong Caribbean cultural ties may be practitioners of an African-based religion even when they only report they are Christian (e.g., Roman Catholic). Show respect to practitioners of these religions, as they may be afraid to disclose this owing to previous prejudice and discrimination from others who condemned them as "primitive" or devil worshippers.

Worship and Devotional Practices

Because these religions pass on their beliefs and practices via oral traditions that may include stories, proverbs, and songs, there is no written sacred scripture. Worship may occur individually, with prayers said in front of an altar that may contain doll-like figures representing deities, glasses with water, rattles, perfumes, oils, and so forth. Incentivizing food or other gifts may be presented to the deity or ancestor spirit when it is petitioned. Altars will vary among traditions, and there may be a separate area for ancestor worship.

Likewise, if spiritism is practiced—that is, the consultation of the dead whose spirits are stuck on earth because of a violent or untoward death—this practice would occur away from where deities and ancestral spirits are venerated. Catholic or other Christian symbols may be present at an altar, depending on the syncretic nature of the practitioner's religiosity.

Practitioners will also seek a priest or priestess for a *consulta* when there is need to request health, protection, or a solution to a problem. The diviner can provide counsel based on the results of a divination. If there is a problem, the priest or priestess will likely instruct the believer to make an offering to remedy the problem. In this way, practitioners can receive physical, emotional, relational, financial, spiritual, and other types of advice and guidance from the deities and their ancestors.

Although there are no formal meeting places, groups may meet for a ceremony or ritual in a private home or outdoor location. These occasions likely will involve singing, drumming, dancing, praying, and other ritual practices. For some religions, each deity may have preferences (e.g., for foods, colors, music) to which the worshipper caters. At these occasions, a priest or priestess may experience altered consciousness or trance. This is believed to involve the emptying of the self and temporary "mounting" or indwelling of a divinity or ancestral spirit; in this way, spiritual entities and ancestors are believed to communicate with humans, and relationships among humans and between humans and spirits can be harmonized. For some, these semidivine beings become accessible only after praying to and honoring ancestral spirits. Some practitioners believe they can communicate with their ancestors and spirit guides through dreams and intuitions. Thus:

- Avoid touching, or only touch with permission and respect, any religious objects the patient may wear or have as an altar at the bedside (e.g., icon, glasses filled with water next to a candle). Never remove a beaded bracelet, necklace, or amulet (religious jewelry). These are viewed as protective.

Illness and Healing: Beliefs and Practices

Illness and premature death are forms of misfortune that can have a variety of sources and causes, including curses, witchcraft, envy, excessive arguing, gossip, and poor decisions. Some illnesses are part of a person's destiny on earth; such people brought this destiny with them, and while there's no way to avoid it, with religious guidance and intervention from the deities, the severity of the illness can be changed. To counter misfortune and be restored to health, a practitioner seeks a priest or priestess who can perform a divination and learn from the deities what ought to be done to restore balance. Some illnesses, however, will be understood as having biological causes, and Western medicine is sought. Indeed, priests or priestesses will counsel devotees to consult a physician and follow prescribed therapies. While the deities will help, the devotees must also help themselves. Thus:

- Patients who are not healed may suffer a spiritual guilt that they have not obeyed or adequately pacified a deity.
- Patients may seek a priest or priestess (or folk healer) initially and regardless of circumstances, or only when there is an inability of Western healthcare to cure.
- If it is determined that one's illness has spiritual causes, the diviner will determine what offering is needed to resolve the problem. This can be an herbal bath; a spiritual cleansing with fruits, vegetables, fish, birds, or other ingredients; or a treatment of an illness through herbal tinctures and infusions. The ingredients used come from ritual knowledge to which only priests or priestesses have access.

Beginning of Life: Beliefs and Practices

Scientific explanations for why pregnancy occurs or does not are understood by those acculturated to Western societies. A curse or witchcraft done to the woman or man to prevent conception, however, may also explain infertility. Infertility concerns may be brought to a priest or priestess, and a ritual performed to remove the witchcraft. The couple would likely then be advised to consult a physician. Pregnant women may take various herbs to foster health. Various rituals may be performed after birth. Thus:

- Assess what prenatal herbs may be taken, and consider their impact.
- When planning the delivery experience, inquire what rituals or hygienic practices may be desired.

End of Life: Beliefs and Practices

Death allows transition from the visible world to an invisible world, where the deceased's spirit continues to exist. Thus, ancestors can watch and inspire the living. Death-related rituals are typically only for the initiated. Prayers and chanting are in lieu of last rites. A body will be buried in the ground, not cremated. Thus:

- When death is imminent, inquire as to how the healthcare team can support the family to observe postmortem practices. The family (or religious community) will want to take the body as soon as possible from the healthcare setting so that ceremonies can take place.
- If an autopsy is required, this will require explanation or negotiation with the family and priest or priestess.

Diet and Lifestyle: Prescriptions and Proscriptions

- Caribbean cultures are collectivist. Thus, accommodating large family visits and sharing healthcare decision making may be necessary.
- Patients in the process of becoming initiates (often evidenced by the wearing of white) may be instructed to observe certain prescriptions and proscriptions for the rest of their lives. For any initiated practitioner, it is important to assess if there are any foods, drinks, or activities that should be avoided.
- Some Rastafarians (or Rastas) smoke marijuana ("ganja") to gain insight. It may be smoked while meditating with members of the faith community (sharing the pipe or "chalice"). Rastas also ban drugs that are abusive and often avoid alcohol, tobacco, and caffeine to not destroy the body—the "temple of God."

Additional Miscellaneous Nursing Implications

- The head is considered by some as the location where the divine interacts with the human. Nurses should ask permission before touching, washing, or treating the crown of the head.
- The color of clothing is sometimes meaningful. For some religions, white represents purity, and black is thought to attract spirits of the dead and is not to be worn. Sheets, blankets, towels, and clothing should be white or light colored.
- The spirits of the dead who experienced a traumatic death (e.g., murder, suicide) are believed to be stuck on earth. These spirits are to be avoided and not talked about, for fear that interaction with them will bring about one's own premature death. Because such deaths often occur in hospitals, a practitioner will not want to visit a hospital for long.
- When clinicians do not share a patient's interpretation of an illness, this discrepancy can contribute to a patient's "noncompliance" with treatment. Clinicians must seek to understand the patient's worldview and negotiate a treatment plan

with the patient as a "therapeutic ally" (Kleinman, Eisenberg, & Good, 1978). Kleinman et al. suggested the following: (a) Openly discuss the discrepant models, encouraging questions; (b) educate the patient if the illness model is thought to be harmful, negotiating a plan; and (c) engage cultural brokers (e.g., family, patient's clergy) if needed.

Ways and Words to Comfort

- Be respectful; do not judge.

Bibliography

Duncan, C. (n.d.). *What's Santería?* Retrieved from http://www.aboutsanteria.com/santeriacutea.html

Kleinman, A., Eisenberg, L., & Good, B. (1978). Culture, illness, and care. *Annals of Internal Medicine, 88*, 251–258. doi:10.7326/0003-4819-88-2-251

Pasquali, E. A. (1994). Santería. *Journal of Holistic Nursing, 12*(4), 380–390. doi:10.1177/089801019401200407

The Pluralism Project. (2018). *Afro-Caribbean traditions.* Harvard University. Retrieved from http://pluralism.org/religions/afro-caribbean/

Rosario, A. M., & De La Rosa, M. (2014). Santería as informal mental health support among U.S. Latinos with cancer. *Journal of Religion & Spirituality in Social Work, 33*(1), 4–18. doi:10.1080/15426432.2014.873294

Tanenbaum Center for Interreligious Understanding. (2009). *The medical manual for religio-cultural competence.* New York, NY: Author.

3

Bahá'í

Other Names and Similar Religious Traditions

None.

Social and Historical Background

In Persia (now Iran), in the early 1800s, a spiritually precocious young man preached that a Promised One would soon come. Although this Divine Teacher (the Báb) and his small following were persecuted and killed, Bahá'u'lláh was inspired by and promulgated the Báb's teachings. This led to his imprisonment, during which he had a vision informing him that he was the Promised One. These prophets are thought to be the most recent divine messengers, with Moses, Buddha, Jesus, Zarathustra, Muhammad, and others being predecessors.

Indeed, the different faith traditions begun by these different prophets are thought to reflect the reality of a oneness of religion, and this reflects the reality that there is a oneness of God (albeit ascribed different names). Bahá'ís believe that all are called to bring about "a unified world," a oneness of humanity. That is, all were created by God in love, all were created as equals, and all persons should strive to be kind to each other and restore this oneness of humanity. Thus, even though the religion began in 1844, gender, racial, and all forms of equality were pursued.

Worship and Devotional Practices

Bahá'ís are expected daily to (a) refine their inner character through devotion (e.g., prayer, meditation, fasting, pilgrimage, reading scripture) and (b) work to transform society (e.g., community service, evangelism)—the work that truly develops spiritual qualities. Although they worship a personal God, collective layperson-led worship, study, and socializing at a "feast" every 19 days is encouraged.

Bahá'u'lláh's writings, or revelations from God, are the sacred scriptures of the Bahá'í faith. His prolific writings are freely available at www.bahai.org/library/authoritative-texts/bahaullah.

Three prayers recorded by Bahá'u'lláh are obligatory. That is, Bahá'ís are to recite one of these three prayers each day: a brief prayer recited between noon and sunset; a medium-length prayer recited morning, noon, and evening that involves washing hands and then face and then bending and sitting while reciting various parts of the prayer; or a long prayer said once a day, with different parts recited while sitting or standing. Prayers are always recited while facing Bahjí, Israel, where the shrine honoring Bahá'u'lláh is located. Thus:

■ Assist the patient, if requested, with obligatory prayer (described earlier). A website for locating the direction of Bahjí is available at https://qiblih.com. The patient may wish for a basin with which to wash hands and face.

Illness and Healing: Beliefs and Practices

Scripture encourages believers to obtain competent healthcare providers to maintain health and holistically treat disease. A fundamental belief in science harmonizing with faith further supports use of modern healthcare practices.

Bahá'ís adopt a very long view of suffering in this world. They understand tests and difficulties as being a sign of God's love and that overcoming difficulty is how the soul grows in this world. Sickness is understood as one of the most difficult tests we are asked to endure in this life.

Beginning of Life: Beliefs and Practices

Because life (and a soul) begins at conception, abortion—unless medically necessary—is strongly discouraged. Breastfeeding is advocated by scripture and science.

End of Life: Beliefs and Practices

The spiritual development obtained in earthly life prepares that soul for advancement toward God in a nonphysical afterlife. Organ donation is a choice. Burial is to be within a 1-hour journey from where death occurred. The body is to be placed in a white cloth shroud.

Embalming is not permitted, unless vital to preserve the body when it cannot be buried soon after death. Teachings urge against cremation. Thus:

- If requested, engage the family (or local Bahá'í community) in preparing the body for burial.
- Ensure that amputated limbs, stillbirths, or donated bodies are disposed of respectfully by burial.

Diet and Lifestyle: Prescriptions and Proscriptions

- Bahá'í religious practices are standardized everywhere throughout the world and overseen by the religion's global governing institution, the Universal House of Justice, located in Haifa, Israel. Purely cultural practices (such as dress) are diverse, of course, and vary according to each country.
- From March 2 to 21, 15- to 70-year-olds fast from sunrise to sunset. Pregnant and ill persons are exempt as well as those traveling away from home.

Additional Miscellaneous Nursing Implications

- Modesty is important. During exams and treatments, be sure to keep the body well covered.
- There are no clergy; respect lay leaders who visit Bahá'í patients as though they were clergy, as they can offer the same comfort. Instead of a ministry, the authority of the religion is vested in elected institutions that govern the affairs of the Bahá'ís.

Ways and Words to Comfort

- "Is there any Remover of difficulties save God? Say: Praised be God! He is God! All are His servants, and all abide by His bidding!" (the Báb, Compilations, *Bahá'í Prayers*, p. 27).
- "Say: God sufficeth all things above all things, and nothing in the heavens or in the earth but God sufficeth. Verily, He is in Himself the Knower, the Sustainer, the Omnipotent" (the Báb, Compilations, *Bahá'í Prayers*, p. 28).
- Other prayers for assistance and healing are available online at http://reference.bahai.org/en/t/c/BP.

Bibliography

Bahá'í International Community. (2018). *The Bahá'í faith*. Retrieved from http://www.bahai.org

Bahá'u'lláh, Báb, & 'Abdu'l-Bahá. (1991). *Bahá'í prayers: A selection of prayers revealed by Bahá'u'lláh, the Báb, and 'Abdu'l-Bahá*. Bahá'í Reference

Library. Baha'I International Community. Retrieved from http://reference .bahai.org/en/t/c/BP/

Davidson, J. E., Boyer, M. L., Casey, D., Matzel, S. C., & Walden, C. D. (2008). Gap analysis of cultural and religious needs of hospitalized patients. *Critical Care Nursing Quarterly, 31*(2), 119–126. doi:10.1097/01.CNQ .0000314472.33883.d4

Kourosh, A., & Hosoda, E. (2007). Eye on religion: The Bahá'í Faith. *Southern Medical Journal, 100*(4), 445–446. doi:10.1097/SMJ.0b013e3180316af3

Metropolitan Chicago Healthcare Council. (2002). *Guidelines for healthcare providers interacting with patients of the Bahá'í religion and their families*. Retrieved from https://www.advocatehealth.com/assets/documents/ faith/cgbahai.pdf

Pereira-Salgado, A., Mader, P., O'Callaghan, C., Boyd, L., & Staples, M. (2017). Religious leaders' perceptions of advance care planning: A secondary analysis of interviews with Buddhist, Christian, Hindu, Islamic, Jewish, Sikh and Bahá'í leaders. *BMC Palliative Care, 16*(1), 79. doi:10.1186/s12904 -017-0239-3

Setrakian, H. V., Rosenman, M. B., & Szucs, K. A. (2011). Breastfeeding and the Bahá'í faith. *Breastfeeding Medicine, 6*(4), 221–225. doi:10.1089/bfm .2010.0098

4

Buddhism

Other Names and Similar Religious Traditions

There are many varieties of Buddhism; indeed, around 200 schools of Buddhism continue. There are three primary branches: **Theravada** or **Southern** (predominant in Southeast Asian cultures); **Mahayana** (prevalent in North and East Asian cultures); and **Vajrayana** or **Tantric** or **Tibetan** (practiced in northern India, Mongolia, and Himalayan countries). Within each of these branches are branches (e.g., **Nicheren**, **Pure Land**, and **Zen** are schools of Buddhism). In North America, Buddhists may be inspired by a hybrid of different branches.

Social and Historical Background

Given these variations that no doubt result from Buddhism's 2,500 years of existence and interpretations in diverse cultures spanning the Asian continent, it is vital to recognize that beliefs and practices differ widely among Buddhists. Generally, however, it is accepted that this religious philosophy began with the enlightenment and teaching of Siddhartha Gautama (i.e., Buddha, "the Awakened Mind"). Buddha's teachings focused on what contributes to suffering and how it can be purged by an awakened mind. Thus, Buddhists strive to achieve an awakened mind or enlightenment, just as the Buddha did. Enlightenment involves gaining insight about the attachments that cause suffering (and ultimately a permanent state of clarity about the nature of reality) and achieving freedom through spiritually releasing oneself. With death, the ultimate freedom, release from being bound to material existence (i.e., *nirvana*) can occur.

These beliefs are identified in the Four Noble Truths of Buddha: (1) all are subject to suffering, (2) suffering is caused by ignorance and attachments to impermanent things, (3) the bondage of attachments will end when one achieves enlightenment, and (4) the way to achieve enlightenment is through the Eightfold Path. The Eightfold Path directs followers to live ethically and develop mental discipline and wisdom by having true or right understanding (knowing Four Noble Truths); thinking (striving for enlightenment); speech (not talking hurtfully); livelihood (abstaining from harmful ways of making a living); behavior (doing good; see Five Precepts); effort (having a compassionate state of mind); concentration (maintaining dispassion for things impermanent); and mindfulness (achieved through intense meditation). Likewise, Buddha's teaching includes Five Precepts, which encompass not taking life, not taking what is not given, not engaging in sexual activity that is hurtful to another, not lying or speaking harshly, and not taking substances that intoxicate the mind. Depending on the branch of Buddhism and whether one is lay or a monk or nun, additional proscriptions may be followed.

Worship and Devotional Practices

The primary spiritual practice for developing an awakened mind is meditation. Although Buddhism does not espouse a salvific, eternal, or sovereign deity, some will pray for special blessings (e.g., healing) to a Buddhist deity. Buddhists often keep a statue of the Buddha or other Buddhist saints and divinities on an altar; these remind them of their aspirations and provide a visual focus during meditation. These statues are found not only at temples, monasteries, and religious centers but also often in one's home. Fresh-cut flowers and incense (or electric lights) as well as other offerings are placed on the altar. Devout Buddhists meditate in the early morning and throughout the day. Organized, regular communal meetings occur at least weekly at a temple or other religious center, where attendees can recite mantras (phrases with special efficacy) and liturgies, meditate, learn about Buddhism, sing devotional songs or chant mantras, experience fellowship, and so forth. These liturgies, mantras, and teachings are found in numerous ancient Buddhist texts; texts used vary among branches of Buddhism. Thus:

- Support meditation or other spiritual practices. Meditation often requires a focus on breathing, so assisting the patient to a conducive posture will be appreciated (e.g., supporting a straight back). Inquire when the patient would like uninterrupted and quiet time, and organize care to accommodate patient wishes. If pertinent, schedule medications that befuddle the mind so that the meditation can occur during their nadir. Of course, consult the patient regarding preferences.
- Often meditation involves focusing on a visual object or on a mantra. Several websites provide Buddhist mantras. One site is WildMind

Buddhist Meditation (www.wildmind.org/mantras/figures), which includes the mantra to the Medicine Buddha, often sought by those who are ill. Recordings are available online.

- Set up the environment to facilitate the spiritual practice as the patient desires. Buddhists may use various objects to enhance their meditation (e.g., recorded meditations, chants, and scriptures; icons or items for visual focus; prayer beads, bell, cymbals, or wheel). With any of these religious objects or any Buddhist text, request permission before handling; treat with utmost respect (e.g., do not lay them on the floor or put things on top of them).

Illness and Healing: Beliefs and Practices

Although a Buddhist will likely accept modern scientific explanations for disease, Buddhist teachings also recognize that immoderate behaviors that disturb a person's balance also contribute to illness (e.g., overeating, intoxication, stress, anger). A lifestyle of moderation in all things is encouraged. Thus:

- Respect a Buddhist patient's desire to maintain a calm emotional state and atmosphere.

Likewise, the path to enlightenment inherently brings health. That is, the Buddha's "Three Marks of Existence" (i.e., that everything is impermanent, that even our self is continually changing and no aspect is permanent, and that nothing has a fixed identity) remind the Buddhist that things of the world do not provide true or lasting happiness; by gaining awareness of one's attachments and releasing them, one lessens suffering and promotes health. Thus:

- Support patients who may want to pursue meditation or other spiritual practices.
- Some may interpret their suffering as resulting from attachment to physical well-being and therefore may be accepting of unnecessary discomfort and shun therapies.

It is also possible for some Buddhists to interpret an illness or disability as the result of previous wrongdoing (in this or a previous life). Therefore, the health challenge is an opportunity to right a wrong, to earn merit by responding to the challenge in a virtuous way. Thus:

- Avoid responses to patients that could convey blame, pity, hopelessness, or frame the patient as a victim. Instead, support interpretations that appreciate illness as a prompt for transformation and an opportunity to model or teach others.
- Respect that some may work to right past wrongs by doing good deeds.

Some branches of Buddhism suggest prayers to deities of healing (e.g., Medicine Buddha) or mantras of purification or specific visualizations and meditations to promote health. These can be offered by Buddhist clergy, the patient, or any other knowledgeable Buddhist. Some may accept folk beliefs that posit that a health challenge results from spirits and request a Buddhist clergy to pacify the spirit. In contrast, some Buddhists believe their bodies are the abode of deities; this belief motivates them to care for their bodies. Thus:

- Facilitate clergy visit if requested (place request with chaplain services, per policy).
- For those who view their bodies as an abode for a deity, let this motivate healthful responses to illness.

Given the Buddha's admonition to not be intoxicated, some may avoid medications that befuddle the mind and instead use meditation to manage pain or other symptoms. Buddhists, however, do accept medications that relieve suffering. Thus:

- When narcotics or other therapeutics that might cloud awareness are prescribed, discuss with the patient how he or she prefers to manage symptom(s), and collaborate to titrate the medication per patient wishes so that clarity of mind and calmness can be balanced. Inform the patient about nonpharmacological methods.

Beginning of Life: Beliefs and Practices

Any contraception that prevents fertilization is acceptable. Beliefs pertaining to abortion and other perinatal decisions are not codified, and decisions will reflect the branch of Buddhism as well as culture of those involved. A couple may seek the council of their clergy if they are faced with an ethical decision.

Likewise, the practices surrounding child birthing vary, reflecting the cultural diversity of Buddhists. Some may provide a name at birth but then change it at a subsequent naming ceremony. Owing to folk beliefs in many Buddhist countries, babies born with a deformity or disability may be viewed as reaping the consequence for a wrong committed in a previous life. Parents of babies that die may want a Buddhist clergy or layperson to conduct a ritual.

End of Life: Beliefs and Practices

Key to end-of-life decisions and practices is the belief that the self is impermanent and in a repeated process of dying and rebirthing (reincarnation). Each life span allows one to achieve more enlightenment and increase the ability to attain nirvana. Life choices, including those right at the end of life, will affect the merit accrued at death (*karma*). However, when there is no clear ethical answer for an end-of-life decision and the intent of the decision maker is good, this is thought to provide balance if indeed the wrong choice is made.

There is no uniform guidance for Buddhists on end-of-life dilemmas. Anything aimed at promoting death (e.g., euthanasia), however, might be viewed as unacceptable. Given Buddhism's emphasis on detachment, it may be less likely that Buddhists opt for technologies that unnaturally prolong life. For those in a persistent vegetative state, Buddhists would agree that compassion should prevail and life be supported, unless a secondary complication requiring medical intervention occurs; when that happens, then aggressive intervention should be withheld.

When such ethical decisions arise, however, some will take guidance solely from the Buddha's precepts, whereas others will give the Buddhist core value of compassion preeminence. Thus:

- For Buddhists at the end of life, assess how beliefs influence their care preferences, as they will vary between differing schools of Buddhism and individual Buddhists within those schools.

When Buddhists are actively dying, they are encouraged to be as calm and meditative as possible. This provides an example for others and may contribute to a better rebirth. Thus:

- Enable the patient to meditate, especially in the final moments (e.g., avoid medications that cloud the mind, play recorded chants if the patient is alone). Ideally, such end-of-life care is planned with the patient beforehand.
- For some, it is vital to have Buddhist clergy and fellow Buddhists present to meditate and chant on behalf of the patient at the time of death and thereafter (until the body is considered fully dead). If needed, a Buddhist chaplain can be located through a directory found at www.buddhistchaplains.org.

Some believe that consciousness can continue to exist in or around the patient's body for up to 3 days after "death." Furthermore, whereas some accept "brain death" as fulfilling the criteria for death, others will require that a skilled Buddhist observer confirm death has occurred when there is no evidence of heat, vitality, and sentience. Thus:

- Given the diversity of Buddhist schools' teachings, assess end-of-life practices that will have pertinence for nursing care (e.g., needs at the time of death, postmortem practices).

Diet and Lifestyle: Prescription and Proscriptions

Given the emphasis on clarity of mind, some may consume intoxicants only in moderation or never. Although many practice vegetarianism, many do not. Food eaten will reflect the patient's culture. The guideline of moderation may influence various aspects of lifestyle. Thus:

- If preferred diet is unknown, provide vegetarian food. Assess diet and other lifestyle preferences when they pertain to health.

Some Buddhists wear cords or amulets around their necks or wrists. Thus:

- Do not remove wearable religious items without patient approval. Treat with respect.

Additional Miscellaneous Nursing Implications

- Remember that even though a Buddhist patient might meditate and remain calm amid suffering, this does not mean the patient is not suffering and feeling the pain of impermanence.

Ways and Words to Comfort

- Facilitate Buddhist clergy visit if requested or if the patient is dying and family verifies it is wanted. If chaplain services are not available to request Buddhist clergy, one can be located via an online directory, Buddhist Chaplains.org (buddhistchaplains.org/cmsms/index.php?page=about-us).
- Support meditation or other devotional practices (see "Worship and Devotional Practices").

Bibliography

Keown, D. (2005). End of life: The Buddhist view. *Lancet, 366,* 952–955. doi:10.1016/S0140-6736(05)67323-0

McCormick, A. J. (2013). Buddhist ethics and end-of-life care decisions. *Journal of Social Work in End-of-Life & Palliative Care, 9,* 209–225. doi:10.1080/15524256.2013.794060

Metropolitan Chicago Healthcare Council. (2003). *Guidelines for healthcare providers interacting with patients of the Buddhist religion and their families.* Retrieved from https://www.advocatehealth.com/assets/documents/faith/cgbuddhist.pdf

Starkey, C. (2018). A focus on: Buddhism. *Community Practitioner, 91*(6), 25–27.

Toneatto, T. (2012). Buddhists. In E. J. Taylor (Ed.), *Religion: A clinical guide for nurses* (pp. 129–136). New York, NY: Springer Publishing.

5

Christianity: Anabaptist-Descended Denominations

Other Names and Similar Religious Traditions

European free churches, also called historic peace churches, include about two dozen small denominations, most of which include the label **Amish**, **Brethren**, **Mennonites**, **Hutterites**, or **Friends** in their name. This chapter will focus on **Anabaptist**-descended traditions: Brethren, Mennonites, and Hutterites. "**Old Order**" or most traditional Amish, Mennonites, and Hutterites, who are known for their horse-and-buggy transport, are also called **Plain People**.

Social and Historical Background

Anabaptists (believers in adult baptism) have 16th century Germanic roots. All continue to share, in varying degrees, the following commonalities: baptism only when one is of an accountable age and wants to join the fellowship, nonviolence and pursuit of peace and justice for all, simplicity and shunning of materialism, and communal living or economic sharing instead of striving for individual wealth. Thus, among the more conservative expressions of these strands of Anabaptists (e.g., Hutterian Brethren, Old Order Mennonites, Amish), you may observe members wearing simple clothing, shunning technology, conscientiously objecting to military service, living in close-knit communities, and avoiding much participation with secular society. Members of the larger Anabaptist-descended groups (e.g., Mennonite Church USA, Church of the Brethren), however, live and believe much like other Protestant Christians today.

Worship and Devotional Practices

Members of these denominations corporately worship weekly on Sundays, except that most Hutterites worship in community twice daily and most Amish every other Sunday. Whereas Hutterites, Mennonites, and Brethren attend churches, Amish worship in homes. The more conservative Anabaptists will refrain from unnecessary work and business on Sundays. Thus:

- Recognize that for those who experience God especially in communal worship, separation from the community of believers may be particularly distressing. Discuss with the patient how this void might be filled.

There are subtle differences in how the Bible is viewed as a sacred text among Anabaptists. Brethren accept the New Testament as the ultimate revelation of God's purposes yet also view the Old Testament scriptures as providing insight. Mennonites and Amish hold more traditional Christian stances regarding the entire Bible as a sacred scripture. The more conservative may prefer the King James Version of the Bible; Amish and Hutterites may read a German version. Thus:

- When requested, obtain or read the sacred text preferred by the patient.
- Free inspirational reading is available: Mennonites' Third Way offers links to free Bible readings, church newsletter, inspirational stories, and so forth on its website: thirdway.com/subscriptions.

Plain People may be most at ease with prayer as a communal, leader-led experience. Thus:

- If an assessment indicates prayer would be welcomed, inquire as to how the patient prefers to pray. Support or join, as appropriate. Although the Plain People may accept a fellow Christian nurse being present during communal prayer, they may not be comfortable with the nurse praying aloud.

Illness and Healing: Beliefs and Practices

Anabaptist-descended groups accept that the purpose of life, and therefore health, is to love God and serve one's neighbor. Thus, one is to care for one's physical and mental health so that it can be used for God's service. Given the sensitivity to the greater good within the community, expensive or life-extending treatment may be rejected, viewed as poor stewardship. In addition to scientific explanations for disease, they will likely understand disease as a consequence of sin—not the patient's private sin but the sin-caused degradation of all creation. Like other Christians, a patient may request an anointing for physical or spiritual need (i.e., after a time for confession, the church leader applies oil to the forehead of the patient and prays for the specified need while laying hands on the patient). Thus:

- When supporting healthcare decision making, appreciate there will be a desire to balance seeking health and stewardship of personal and societal resources. (A "you're worth it" statement would be inappropriate.)

While there are no unique health-related beliefs or practices of mainstream Mennonites and Brethren, there are numerous distinctions regarding health among Plain People. These unique practices reflect not only fundamental beliefs about relying on God—the ultimate Healer—for all things but also not being worldly and staying to themselves in a communal structure, living simply, and avoiding modern technologies (hence, the agrarian culture). Health behaviors are often explained by these beliefs as well as the resulting pragmatic challenges like cost (as they do not participate in commercial or government insurance programs); low level of formal education (usually not past the eighth grade or age 15); language (English is a second language learned only at school); and difficulty traveling (as they prefer horse and buggy and live rurally). Thus:

- Given the low health literacy and education, avoid medical jargon and language that is complex; use pictures, demonstrations, and role modeling.
- Understand that there is high use of complementary therapies and folk remedies (e.g., herbs, chiropractors, supplements, natural poultices) and delayed entry to any secular healthcare system. Assess for natural remedies that may interfere with treatment plans.

Beginning of Life: Beliefs and Practices

Plain People's midwives typically assist them to give birth at home or in birthing clinics they operate. Likewise, prenatal care (especially first trimester) is often minimal, yet Cesarean rates and low birth weights are no worse than those found among "English" (non-Plain People) in their area. Given their Anabaptist heritage, they do not baptize infants.

They object to contraception, and the average number of births among Plain People is seven to eight per woman. Thus, even though they likely will marry and give birth in their early 20s, they may still be childbearing 15 to 20 years later. Indeed, this explains the exponential population growth among Plain People.

Plain People will also refuse any genetic testing, even though there is a high probability for their offspring to have an inherited disease (given the centuries of consanguineous marriages). The Amish, Mennonite, and Hutterite Genetic Disorder Database kept at www.biochemgenetics.ca/plainpeople/index.php can provide specific analysis of risks by family trees. No testing is believed necessary, given that all children are gifts from God; an abortion would be unthinkable.

Plain People have very low immunization rates. This is not because of religious beliefs necessarily; Kettunen, Nemecek, and Wenger (2017) found that concerns about safety and adverse reactions were barriers for 84 Amish parents in Ohio. They feared receiving multiple vaccines at once would overwhelm the immune system of their children. Thus:

- When discussing immunizations with Plain People, assess for barriers and address those (e.g., consider an altered scheduling). If there is resistance, it may be helpful to appeal to their fundamental belief in living for the good of others.
- When providing prenatal care, remember the local midwife may not be licensed, transportation may involve considerable distance by horse and buggy, and English and health literacy are likely poor.

End of Life: Beliefs and Practices

Mennonites, Brethren, and the Plain People believe in an afterlife (either immediately entering into God's presence at death or doing so after a future resurrection). These Anabaptist-descended groups do believe in a final judgment of the living and the dead; those who have rejected the love of God will not live in the eternal reign of God.

Plain People prefer to care for their elders and the dying at home. Elders will often forgo life-extending therapies so as to not create a financial burden on their family and community. Funerary customs include embalming, returning the body to the home where visitors are received for a couple days prior to the funeral. Women are buried in the white cape in which they were married. The community is actively engaged in funeral preparations, which include hosting and feeding large numbers of people as well as digging the grave by hand.

Diet and Lifestyle: Prescriptions and Proscriptions

For Anabaptist-descended groups (including Plain People), use of tobacco is rare. Amish men who do use tobacco generally chew tobacco or smoke a cigar. There is diversity of thought regarding alcohol; while for some it is sinful, for others moderate drinking (avoiding drunkenness) is acceptable. The diet of Plain People is dominated by starches, sugars, and fats. The cardiovascular effects of the diet, however, may be offset by the considerable physical activities of farming or domesticity.

The lifestyle of Plain People is guided by the New Testament admonition "to keep oneself unspotted from the world" (James 1:27). This is interpreted to mean to not do what the "world" does (e.g., not drive cars, use electricity or a telephone). A dialect of German is spoken in the home; English is learned when one goes to school. Children attend a school taught by one of their own; the equivalent of a formal sixth- to eighth-grade education is typically achieved. Conservative clothing is worn; women wear bonnets, and married men have beards. Thus:

- When planning patient education, prescriptions, or other treatments for Plain People, keep in mind they may not use electrical appliances, telephones, refrigerators, automobiles, indoor plumbing, or anything with a motor. Assess, however, as some may have and use these technologies—especially when caring for the sick or injured. Negotiate with them what is best.
- When a member of an Old Order community does telephone a healthcare provider, know that this may indicate a serious issue and/or that access to the telephone may be very limited; take the call immediately.
- Plan discharge well in advance so that transportation can be arranged.

Additional Miscellaneous Nursing Implications

- Remember there are thousands of communities in which Plain People live; each district is governed by its own rules and customs.
- Modesty is very important for Plain People. Closely guard a patient's privacy (e.g., keep door closed), and allow patients to wear their own clothing if possible. Similarly, provide same-gender nurses as much as possible.
- Respect the need for Plain women to wear their head covering or prayer veiling (known by outsiders as a "bonnet"). They wear these especially when around men, even those within their own family. If a woman wearing a prayer veiling undergoes a procedure (e.g., MRI) where the metal clip keeping the prayer veiling in place needs to be removed, explain this with sensitivity.
- Several Mennonite and Brethren denominations have organizations created to offer various health-related services (e.g., developmental disability services, mental health services,

and retirement and nursing home care). Visit the Mennonite Health Services (MHS) Alliance (www.mhsonline.org) or Anabaptist Disabilities Network (www.adnetonline.org). Local congregations also often organize themselves to provide support for members.

- Plain People take seriously the call to bear others' burdens within the community. They also do not want to engage with the "world." Thus, many do not buy commercial health insurance and are exempt from participating in Medicare, Social Security, and healthcare exchanges. To pay for healthcare costs, many pay with personal cash, and depending on the expense and need, the community pays the rest. The community funds may result from a collection taken on behalf of the patient and/or from the community's "mutual aid" program. Some Amish may have a form of insurance. Regardless, this contributes to the reticence to pay for preventive dental and healthcare, life-extending care, or any expensive care. Amish are therefore very careful consumers, using funds primarily for emergencies and significant concerns. Thus:
  - Provide care as efficiently and economically as possible (e.g., provide as much care in one visit as possible). Avoid allowing nursing students and others in training to provide care, as Plain People expect quality for their cash payment.
  - Negotiate what care they do want. Be sensitive to the reality that decision making may require input from not only family but also church leaders who would be determining financial support.
  - Contact social service, if necessary, to identify free sources of healthcare.
- Among Plain People, men are designated decision makers; thus, healthcare decisions will be made by them (as well as religious leaders if financial support is needed).
- Among Plain People, a stoic response to pain is typical, even in children; educate about how symptom management promotes healing. Plain People may also appear reserved and show no affection in public.

Ways and Words to Comfort

- For Plain People, facilitate connection with one's community (e.g., create space and time for visitors); indeed, the whole family may be present given there are no transportation issues.
- Old Order denominations each have their own hymn book. Encouraging the practitioner to recite a favorite memorized hymn or read from the hymnal will likely comfort.

- Biblical passages particularly comforting include Romans 8:37–39 (about the love of God); John 14:1–6 and Psalm 23 (especially when near death); and the Lord's Prayer as found in Matthew 6:9–13 (see the appendix).
- For Anabaptist-descended groups, traditional Christian comforts are appropriate (see Chapter 21).

Bibliography

Amish Studies/The Young Center. (n.d.). *Health*. Retrieved from https://groups.etown.edu/amishstudies/cultural-practices/health

Church of the Brethren. (n.d.). *About us*. Retrieved from http://www.brethren.org/about

Cleveland Clinic Office of Diversity. (2017). Amish patients. *Diversity Toolkit*. Retrieved from https://my.clevelandclinic.org/-/scassets/files/org/about/diversity/2016-diversity-toolkit.ashx

Hutterites.org. (n.d.). *Hutterian brethren*. Retrieved from http://www.hutterites.org

Kettunen, C., Nemecek, J., & Wenger, O. (2017). Evaluation of low immunization coverage among the Amish population in rural Ohio. *American Journal of Infection Control, 45*(6), 630–634. doi:10.1016/j.ajic.2017.01.032

Kotva, J. J., Jr. (2012). Anabaptist-descended groups: Amish, Brethren, Hutterites, and Mennonites. In E. J. Taylor (Ed.), *Religion: A clinical guide for nurses* (pp. 101–108). New York: Springer.

Mennonite Church USA. (n.d.). *We are Mennonites*. Retrieved from http://mennoniteusa.org/who-we-are

Rohrer, K., & Dundes, L. (2016). Sharing the load: Amish healthcare financing. *Healthcare, 4*(4), 92. doi:10.3390/healthcare4040092

Weller, G. E. R. (2017). Caring for the Amish: What every anesthesiologist should know. *Anesthesia & Analgesia, 124*(5), 1520–1528. doi:10.1213/ane.0000000000001808

6

Christianity: Anglican and Episcopal

Other Names and Similar Religious Traditions

In the United Kingdom, the Anglican church is the Church of England (CoE). Outside the United Kingdom, denominations within the Anglican Communion will have the word Anglican or Episcopal within them. Because these are Christian denominations, see Chapter 21 for further information about nursing implications.

Social and Historical Background

Christianity was introduced to the British Isles beginning in the 2nd century (Common Era). After about a millennium of papal (Roman Catholic) authority, King Henry VIII's anger at the Roman church's refusal to grant an annulment and the Protestant Reformation converged to birth the CoE. British colonialism spread the faith abroad, including to North America. After the United States established independence, the **Episcopal** tradition formalized. Subsequently, a few iterations have been created: the **Reformed Episcopal Church** organized in 1873 to reform what was viewed as a liberalizing denomination; the **Anglican Catholic Church**, as well as several other very small denominations, organized after the Episcopal church began ordaining women as priests in 1976; the **Anglican Church of North America** (founded in 2009) split off largely in reaction to the mother church's recognition of same-sex unions and ordination of homosexual bishops in committed life partnerships; and the **International Communion of the Charismatic Episcopal Church** (ICCEC), a joining of persons from several mainstream Protestant denominations, organized in 1992 to have a denomination that emphasizes not only liturgy (sacraments, or holy acts that reflect outwardly the inward spiritual experience) and the Bible but also the Holy Spirit (i.e., the "power of Pentecost"). Except for the ICCEC, Anglican and Episcopal churches around the world are united as members of the Anglican Communion.

Worship and Devotional Practices

The Anglican/Episcopal (A/E) churches observe liturgical traditions. That is, corporate worship is a central and formalized aspect. Worship will involve Bible readings that are set out in a lectionary (schedule of prescribed passages for each day of the year). These readings, as well as formal prayers, psalms, and various statements of belief, are found in the *Book of Common Prayer* (*BCP*). Anglican *BCP*s around the world are designed to reflect the language and culture of the local believers. Furthermore, most A/E denominations have their own version of the *BCP*, which can be obtained freely online. Thus:

- A/Es are at ease with written or memorized prayers (including the Psalms).
- Assist, as necessary, the patient to read the appropriate *BCP* morning and/or evening passage for the day (e.g., ask the patient what version is preferred, print out the reading, ask a volunteer to read to the patient). Online locations are as follows:
  - Episcopalians: https://www.episcopalchurch.org/page/book -common-prayer (can download it in English, Spanish, or French)
  - Reformed Episcopal: www.recus.org/resources.html (can download original or modern version)
  - Charismatic Episcopal Church: https://www.iccec.org/ prayerandreadings/Prayer-Individual
  - The Anglican Church of North America: will be publishing a *BCP* soon

A/Es meet every Sunday and on major holy days for worship. For baptized members, worship will include participation in Holy Eucharist (communion). Thus:

- A patient missing the religious nurture of church attendance may want to read/have read a short "sermon" available from the Episcopal Church website: episcopaldigitalnetwork.com/ stw/2018/05/22/bible-study-pentecost-4-b-june-17-2018.
- See Chapter 21 for nursing implications of communion.

Illness and Healing: Beliefs and Practices

A/E priests or trained deaconesses offer a special rite (or unction) for healing that includes praying, laying on of hands, and anointing with oil; it is called Ministration to the Sick (see Chapter 21).

Beginning of Life: Beliefs and Practices

Baptism represents becoming the adopted child of God. Although any baptized Christian may baptize another person in a life-threatening circumstance, it is usual to be baptized by a priest. A stillborn or dead infant can be baptized, but it is not considered necessary. There are no other distinctions from other mainstream Christians (see Chapter 21).

End of Life: Beliefs and Practices

There are no distinctions from other mainstream Christians (see Chapter 21). The *BCP* contains special rites for those at the end of life (i.e., Special Ministration at Time of Death, The Rite of Reconciliation). Absolution is pronounced only by a priest or bishop. If none is available, another Christian may state a declaration of forgiveness.

Diet and Lifestyle: Prescriptions and Proscriptions

Lent, the 40 days between Ash Wednesday and Easter Sunday, is a season of reflection and repentance. Holy Week, the week before Easter, is also a special part of Lent. To facilitate reflection and repentance, members are encouraged, but not commanded, to observe a fast. For example, someone might fast from a certain food (e.g., desserts, meats) or simplify their diet. Additionally, the A/Es on the more Catholic end of the spectrum may fast to a certain extent every Friday.

Additional Miscellaneous Nursing Implications

- The desire for a healing ritual will vary. Rituals include Ministration to the Sick (praying, laying on of hands, anointing with oil) and Holy Eucharist (or communion). These rituals can be performed by a priest (also known as vicar or rector) or deacon or deaconess, or Eucharistic Visitor. Ask your chaplaincy service to coordinate this visit; if there is no chaplain service, contact the patient's preferred local A/E church. The patient may be particularly eager for a visitor from the church on Sundays.
- Parish resources may include lay or professionally trained persons who provide physical and/or emotional support: Stephen Ministers, deaconesses, and parish nurses.

Ways and Words to Comfort

- The *BCP* includes a section for "Daily Office" (which includes "Daily Devotions for Individuals and Families") and a section for "Prayers and Thanksgivings" (which includes "Prayers for

Family and Personal Life") (see the earlier section "Worship and Devotional Practices"). Reading a prayer, psalm, or other passage appropriate to the patient situation may be comforting. The *BCP* also contains a section entitled "Prayers for the Sick" with situation-specific prayers (e.g., sick child, before an operation). There are even prayers for nurses!

■ Websites with short A/E prayers exist. Here is a modernization of a prayer offered by ConnectUS (Ayres, 2016) that would be appropriate for any illness: "God, you are the strength of the weak, and the comfort of sufferers. Be merciful and give to [patient's name] your powerful help. May his/her illness become health, and his/her sorrow become joy, through Jesus Christ our Lord. Amen." Similarly, Grace Cathedral (2016) offers "Prayers for Difficult Times." These include prayers for loss of memory, pain, confinement, loss of a child, comfort, and so forth.
An A/E online source for prayers is *The Cradle of Prayer* (2015), available at cradleofprayer.org/this-weeks-prayers.

■ The "Lord's Prayer" is known by any A/E; a recitation or listening to a musical version (e.g., YouTube) will also provide comfort, as it provides the exemplar prayer given by Jesus (Matthew 6:9–13).

■ Contemplative and centering prayer is now more common for laypeople. See www.Contemplativeoutreach.org for more information. A patient can be invited to meditatively pray a short phrase or word repetitively to find comfort or quiet the soul.

Bibliography

Anglican Church in North America. (2019). *About*. Retrieved from http://anglicanchurch.net/?/main/page/about-acna

Ayres, C. (2016). *16 Good Episcopal prayers for the sick*. Retrieved from https://connectusfund.org/16-good-episcopal-prayers-for-the-sick

Church Hymnal Corporation. (n.d.) *The (online) book of common prayer*. Retrieved from https://www.bcponline.org

Church Publishing and Morehouse Church (2005). *Ministry with the sick*. New York, NY: Church Publishing.

The Domestic and Foreign Missionary Society. (2018). *Sermons that work*. Retrieved from http://episcopaldigitalnetwork.com/stw/2018/05/22/bible-study-pentecost-4-b-june-17-2018

The Episcopal Church. (2018). *About us*. Retrieved from https://www.episcopalchurch.org/

Gortner, D. T. (2012). *Anglicans and Episcopalians*. In E. J. Taylor (Ed.), *Religion: A clinical guide for nurses* (pp. 109–116). New York, NY: Springer Publishing.

Grace Cathedral. (n.d.). *Prayers for difficult times*. Retrieved from https://www.gracecathedral.org/prayers-difficult-times

Griswold, F. T. (2009). *Praying our days: A guide and companion*. New York, NY: Morehouse.

International Communion of the Charismatic Episcopal Church. (2018). *About us*. Retrieved from https://www.iccec.org/about-us

The Reformed Episcopal Church. (n.d.). *An overview of the REC*. Retrieved from http://www.recus.org/about.html

7

Christianity: Baptist

Other Names and Similar Religious Traditions

With only a couple of small exceptions, the nearly two dozen Baptist denominations include the word Baptist in their name. The largest denominations include the American Baptists, Southern Baptists, National Baptist Conventions, and the offshoots Cooperative Baptist Fellowship, National Missionary Baptist Convention, and Progressive National Baptist Convention. Because three of these conventions of Baptists are primarily African American, they will be discussed in Chapter 8. The Baptist Worldwide Alliance includes dozens of Baptist conventions from around the world.

Social and Historical Background

The Baptist denomination began in the early 17th century in the Netherlands by a former Church of England minister, who believed that the sacrament of baptism should entail complete water immersion. Baptists were distinguished, in part, from many other Christians by the belief emphasizing a separation of church and state and the need for people to be able to attend whatever church they desired—both in sharp contradiction to the early practices of the Church of England. Baptists also deemed that believers are "competent" to interpret the Bible and responsible for their own personal relationship with God. Baptists were some of the earliest immigrants to the Massachusetts Bay Colony, and they established the first Baptist church in Rhode Island in 1638. Given Baptists' emphasis on evangelism, it is unsurprising that they constitute the largest of Protestant traditions in the United States today. Because they believe each congregation should govern itself rather autonomously, they affiliate loosely with like-minded Baptists in a "convention."

Thus, there is no central doctrinal authority for Baptists; this results in a range of interpretations or beliefs. During the mid-1800s, Baptists in the United States split into a northern (now the American) convention and the Southern Baptist Convention because of differences in beliefs regarding slavery. Today, these two conventions are not differentiated by views on slavery; however, Southern Baptists are more conservative than American Baptists in their interpretations of the Bible and stands on social issues. Furthermore, Baptists around the world will differ somewhat. For example, British Baptists differ from Southern Baptists in their acceptance of women as clergy and their concern for freedom of belief, social justice, and the environment.

Worship and Devotional Practices

Acknowledging Jesus as God's son and inviting him into one's life as Lord and Savior (i.e., "being saved" or "born again") is fundamental. Bible reading, sincere prayer, and fellowship with other believers sustain the believer's relationship with God. Baptists pray without following a prayer book; their prayers are often conversational and spontaneous but may be read. Thus:

- Support prayer or devotional/private worship time (see Chapter 21 for further information).
- Crosswalk.com (n.d.) contains numerous devotionals and links to numerous favorite Baptist pastors' websites (e.g., Max Lucado, Chuck Swindoll, Rick Warren) where there are written and recorded versions of devotionals and prayers. Some are in Spanish.

Illness and Healing: Beliefs and Practices

Most hold views of illness and healing that are akin to those described in Chapter 21. Occasionally, however, a Baptist may believe that God may grant a miraculous healing in response to fervent prayers. With such a belief, it is possible that some will refuse a do-not-resuscitate order so that God can perform a miracle (see "End of Life: Beliefs and Practices.")

When sick, believers often desire prayer. Some will additionally ask for "the laying on of hands" or anointing with oil (see Chapter 21). Although ministers and deacons typically do it, a layperson could also perform this healing ritual for which there is no uniform practice.

Beginning of Life: Beliefs and Practices

Beliefs and practices regarding beginning of life are similar to those of most Christians (see Chapter 21). Of course, there is no infant baptism but rather a service of dedication. There is variation in stances regarding abortion; whereas more conservatives will argue the fetus is to be protected regardless of circumstances of conception, others regard the autonomy of the person making the decision. All, however, will agree that utmost respect for life and for sexuality (within a same-sex marriage) is essential.

End of Life: Beliefs and Practices

Beliefs about what occurs after death are varied. All believe that if the patient was "saved," the patient will have a heavenly, eternal life with God. Some believe that if the patient did not confess Jesus to be Savior (i.e., become saved), then the patient would go to a literal hell. With such a belief, it is not surprising that some family members will fervently attempt to bring their loved one to profess faith. Other Baptists, however, may hold some doubt regarding a hell and accept that God is merciful beyond human understanding. Baptists are free to determine whether to donate an organ and whether to be buried or cremated. Thus:

- For family members praying for a miracle when healthcare professionals have exhausted treatment options, referral to a chaplain or Baptist clergy will be important.
- If no spiritual care expert is available, nurse responses that may be helpful will include nonjudgmental empathy and naming the family's wishes and logic (e.g., "If I understand correctly, the family is anxious about Mom dying and is praying that God will create a miracle to extend her life") and exploring what "miracle" means (e.g., "What's the miracle that you're hoping for?"). Based on the patient/family's response, the nurse can determine further responses (Shinall, Stahl, & Bibler, 2018):
  - If the wish for a miracle reflects a straddling of denial and acceptance, the nurse can gently support this cognitive processing by not challenging the denial mechanism.
  - If the lack of a miracle is shaking one's faith, then using a therapeutic presence to allow the patient to listen to self will be helpful.
  - If the prayer for a miracle comes from an integrated, well-developed faith and it contrasts with the healthcare provider's worldview, then that needs to be respectfully acknowledged.

Diet and Lifestyle: Prescriptions and Proscriptions

There are no dietary directives. Although today there is variation in whether to abstain or not from alcohol and tobacco, traditionally it was shunned.

Additional Miscellaneous Nursing Implications

■ Some congregations have caregiving teams that mobilize when members assigned to them experience crises, like hospitalization. These may be a resource for patients.

Ways and Words to Comfort

■ Most Baptists would gratefully receive an offer of prayer from a nurse. They would be used to a colloquial style of prayer (see Chapter 21).

■ Baptist patients who ask a nurse to read from the Bible would be likely to want to hear a psalm, a story about Jesus's healing ministry (found in Matthew, Mark, Luke, or John), or a book (epistle) attributed to the Apostle Paul (e.g., Romans, Galatians, Ephesians).

■ Baptists love hymns, gospel songs, and African American spirituals; singing or playing such music would likely be therapeutic.

Bibliography

American Baptist Churches USA. (n.d.). *Our history*. Retrieved from http://www.abc-usa.org/what_we_believe/our-history

Association of Religion Data Archives. (n.d.). *Baptist family*. Retrieved from http://www.thearda.com/denoms/families/trees/familytree_baptist.asp

Clark, P. Y. (2012). *Baptists*. In E. J. Taylor (Ed.), *Religion: A clinical guide for nurses* (pp. 123–128). New York, NY: Springer Publishing.

Cooperative Baptist Fellowship. (n.d.). *About*. Retrieved from http://www.cbf.net/about

Crosswalk.com. (n.d.). *Devotionals*. Retrieved from https://www.crosswalk.com/devotionals

Shinall, M. C., Jr., Stahl, D., & Bibler, T. M. (2018). Addressing a patient's hope for a miracle. *Journal of Pain & Symptom Management, 55*(2), 535–539. doi:10.1016/j.jpainsymman.2017.10.002

Southern Baptist Convention. (n.d.). *About us*. Retrieved from http://www.sbc.net/aboutus

World Council of Churches. (n.d.). *Baptist churches*. Retrieved from https://www.oikoumene.org/en/church-families/baptist-churches

8

Christianity: Historically Black Denominations

Other Names and Similar Religious Traditions

African American Christianity is not a denomination but rather a categorization of several Christian denominations that share an African American cultural distinctiveness. These denominations include those of Baptist traditions (i.e., National Baptist Conventions and the offshoots National Missionary Baptist Convention, National Baptist Church of America, Inc., and the Progressive National Baptist Convention); African Methodist Episcopal (AME) and AME Zion; and the Pentecostal denominations of Church of God in Christ, Pentecostal Assemblies of the World, and Full Gospel Baptist Fellowship. Although most Black Christians in the United States are members of a Protestant denomination, a national survey observed 6% identified as Roman Catholic (Taylor, Chatters, & Brown, 2014).

Social and Historical Background

Whereas some historically Black denominations arose as parallel churches to segregated White churches, others evolved because of disagreements with the parent denomination. Regardless, these denominations have strong roots within the Black communities they serve and play a central role in the lives of their members. Indeed, Blacks attend church more often and have higher levels of spirituality and religiosity than non-Latino Whites. Blacks who are female, married, older, and from the South are the most religious (Taylor et al., 2014).

To further appreciate the importance of religiosity for Blacks, it is important to remember the long history of enslavement as well as modern abuses such as the Tuskegee experiment. These power imbalances have contributed to lower levels of education and income, increased incarceration and domestic violence, difficulty with and fear about accessing health, and so forth; the consequences include health disparities between Blacks and non-Latino Whites. Given this social history, it may not be surprising that Blacks often use their religious beliefs and practices to cope with health challenges. Indeed, high religiosity/spirituality is associated with lower all-cause mortality and psychosocial morbidity among Blacks (e.g., Cheadle et al., 2015; Oates, 2016).

Worship and Devotional Practices

Although the theology of historically Black denominations differs minimally from the Protestant streams of Christianity from which they emerged, their worship style and emphasis on living the gospel message through social justice do. The individual believer frequently uses colloquial prayer and songs to communicate with and praise God and find comfort and guidance. More educated Black Christians may read the Bible and spiritual materials, whereas those who are less educated are more apt to seek religious support by watching religious television programs. See Chapter 21 for nursing implications.

Illness and Healing: Beliefs and Practices

See Chapter 21 or the chapters on Baptists, Pentecostalism, or Methodists, as appropriate to the patient's denomination.

Beginning of Life: Beliefs and Practices

See Chapter 21 or the chapters on Baptists, Pentecostalism, or Methodists, as appropriate to the patient's denomination.

End of Life: Beliefs and Practices

See Chapter 21 or the chapters on Baptists, Pentecostalism, or Methodists, as appropriate to the patient's denomination.

Diet and Lifestyle: Prescriptions and Proscriptions

See Chapter 21 or the chapters on Baptists, Pentecostalism, or Methodists, as appropriate to the patient's denomination.

Additional Miscellaneous Nursing Implications

See Chapter 21 or the chapters on Baptists, Pentecostalism, or Methodists, as appropriate to the patient's denomination.

- Health promotion and education are feasible and successful in Black Christian churches if lay leaders are actively engaged in the process.
- Some Black churches will recruit nurses to assist ushers during church services; they may potentially be of assistance as lay health workers for non–African American nurses interested in providing community-based health services.
- Given the import of spirituality and religion in the lives of Blacks, this fundamental orientation can be tapped to improve health promotion. Appeal to "the body as a temple." An effective brochure framed breast cancer screening in this way: "You are not given the spirit of fear but of power over your health. Visiting a medical professional does not mean you lack faith—it means you are acting on your faith" (Best, Spencer, Friedman, Hall, & Billings, 2016, p. 622).

Ways and Words to Comfort

- Black Christians emphasize "blessings" rather than "good luck." Listen for this and mirror the language and behavior as appropriate.
- Reminders of the powerfulness and lovingness of God to heal (e.g., "He's got the whole world in His hands, including you and me, sister").
- Words or recordings of spirituals and gospel songs.
- If assessed as appropriate and noncoercive, offer to pray (see Chapter 21).

Bibliography

Best, A. L., Spencer, S. M., Friedman, D. B., Hall, I. J., & Billings, D. (2016). The influence of spiritual framing on African American women's mammography intentions: A randomized trial. *Journal of Health Communication, 21*(6), 620–628. doi:10.1080/10810730.2015.1114055

Cheadle, A. C., Dunkel Schetter, C., Gaines Lanzi, R., Reed Vance, M., Sahadeo, L. S., & Shalowitz, M. U. (2015). Spiritual and religious resources in African American women: Protection from depressive symptoms after childbirth. *Clinical Psychological Science, 3*(2), 283–291. doi:10.1177/2167702614531581

Hamilton, J. B., Moore, A. D., Johnson, K. A., & Koenig, H. G. (2013). Reading *The Bible* for guidance, comfort, and strength during stressful life events. *Nursing Research, 62*(3), 178–184. doi:10.1097/NNR.0b013e31828fc816

Lindner, E. W. (Ed.). (2010). *Yearbook of American and Canadian churches*. Nashville, TN: Abington. Retrieved from https://www.cokesbury.com/digitalstore/subscription/9780687466863.pdf

Progressive National Baptist Convention. (n.d.). *History of the PNBC*. Retrieved from http://www.pnbc.org/History

Oates, G. L. (2016). Effects of religiosity dimensions on physical health across non-elderly Black and White American panels. *Review of Religious Research, 58*(2), 249–270. doi:10.1007/s13644-015-0239-9

Taylor, R. J., Chatters, L. M., & Brown, R. K. (2014). African American religious participation. *Review of Religious Research, 56*(4), 513–538. doi:10.1007/s13644-013-0144-z

9

Christianity: Jehovah's Witness

Other Names and Similar Religious Traditions

Several legal corporations in various countries are used to supporting the preaching and teaching of Jehovah's Witnesses. The primary
legal entity in the United States is the Watch Tower Bible & Tract
Society of Pennsylvania (2018). Related nonprofits in other countries
will often have Watchtower or Watch Tower in their names.

Social and Historical Background

In Pennsylvania in the late 1800s, a group began studying the Bible
to compare its teachings with what Christian churches were teaching.
They concluded there were differences and began publishing their
findings in the *Watchtower—Announcing Jehovah's Kingdom*. This
magazine continues to be a prime way that Jehovah's Witnesses (JWs)
share their teachings, as members often distribute it door to door and
through their official international website (jw.org). Although only
men assume leadership positions in the church, all are considered
ministers; there are no paid clergy.

Worship and Devotional Practices

Jehovah is God, and Jesus is God's son. Jehovah God is approached
via Jesus Christ, who gave his redemptive sacrifice for humanity.
JWs convene twice a week in Kingdom Halls to worship and study.
Likewise, they are encouraged to worship as a family once a week.
JWs' scripture is the Bible (the *New World Translation of the Holy
Scriptures*, completed by JW scholars, is their preferred translation
of the Bible); they believe that the Bible is inerrant and interpret it
literally unless the passage is clearly meant to be metaphorical. The

decisions of a JW are to always be made in alignment with Biblical teaching. If the Bible does not provide a directive, then it is up to the believer to prayerfully consider what is right based on his or her understanding of Bible principles. Thus:

- JWs prefer reading the *New World Translation* of the Bible (available online at www.jw.org/en/publications/bible/study-bible/books). If it is not available, other respected versions of the Bible are acceptable.
- JWs typically approach worship through Bible study. Bible study guides are available on the jw.org website and in *The Watchtower*.

JWs observe only one holy day, the Memorial, which commemorates the Lord's Evening Meal (Last Supper of Jesus just prior to his death). Thus, JWs have communion only once a year on a day near the Jewish Passover. Indeed, the veneration of any other symbolism of religion, nationality, or secular culture that is used in worship is viewed as idolatrous and pagan. Thus:

- Christian holidays (e.g., Christmas), national holidays, and birthdays are not celebrated.
- Avoid presenting JWs with icons such as flags or national emblems; pictures of Jesus, superstars, or other idols; cross-shaped objects (including flowers arranged in these shapes).

Illness and Healing: Beliefs and Practices

JWs believe that illness and disability (physical or emotional) are not imposed by God but rather are the result of various factors such as heredity, lifestyle choices, the environment, and other accepted causes. However, they do give considerable weight to Bible principles and refer to their religious publications in coping with illness or for help in making decisions regarding healthcare. If there is no clear Bible principle involved, then it is a matter of personal choice. Although JWs state they do not believe in "faith healing" and they readily seek modern healthcare and accept most treatments, it is possible that some may believe they need to seek God's guidance and support in prayer along with persistent effort (especially with mental health challenges and addictions). Thus:

- When discussing a treatment plan, it is important to assess whether the JW believes it to be in accord with Bible teaching. Keep in mind that such discussion will be difficult for patients if they think you do not respect their beliefs.
- A patient who is uncertain about what the Bible or church teaches may want to consult with a JW expert (e.g., local leader, Hospital

Liaison Committee member). Fear of making a wrong decision may reflect the possibility of damaging his or her relationship with Jehovah God.

In healthcare, what JWs are most known for is their refusal to receive blood. This directive is based on Biblical commands (primarily in Acts 15:28–29 but also in Mosaic laws). Thus, receiving blood or other body parts (or eating animal meat that is not properly bled) is forbidden. Thus:

- JWs abstain from whole blood or any of the primary components (i.e., blood, red blood cells, white blood cells, platelets, or plasma).
- Because the Bible does not directly address blood fractions (e.g., hemoglobin, interferons, clotting factors, albumin), JWs may base a decision to receive these on their own conscience.
- Organ donation and transplantation is another personal choice; if an organ is accepted, most of the blood must be removed.
- Blood or the primary blood components that have been stored, even if autologous, likewise are forbidden (e.g., preoperative blood donation). Some JWs, however, will accept tests or treatments involving withdrawal of their blood for reinfusing after being tagged or mixed with a therapeutic agent.
- Nonblood medical alternatives, medicines, and surgical techniques used in place of blood transfusion are acceptable. Autotransfusion techniques (e.g., cell salvage) are a personal choice. Likewise, use of a heart–lung machine primed with nonblood fluids, hemodialysis without a blood prime, and hemodilution are all for the JW patient to conscientiously decide.
- Because of the potential for legal sequelae, most JWs carry on their person an advance medical directive release document (a wallet-sized card). When admitting a JW to a healthcare institution, that institution may have additional documentation to complete.
- Given the complexity of medical options and how these may be viewed by JWs, contact the local Hospital Liaison Committee member or the Department of Hospital Information Services at the JW headquarters, available 24/7 at 718-560-4300 (United States) or +1-718-560-4700 (international). Or visit the JW.org website page for medical professionals at www.jw.org/en/medical-library/hospital-liaison-committee-hlc-contacts/united-states.
- After analysis or discharge of any JW's blood and tissues (e.g., placenta), dispose of them; never use or donate them for other purposes.

- If a court orders a blood transfusion for a JW (or his or her child), appreciate that this could be viewed as medical rape. Serious physiological and spiritual damage may result to the Witness patient, or any patient for that matter, whose clear wishes regarding strongly held beliefs are ignored, whether by a healthcare provider, close relative, or court of law.
- Above all, communicate with the patient (or parents) to provide mutually acceptable care. JWs do vary in what they believe is acceptable to their conscience. Hold their decision, if it runs counter to church admonitions, in strictest confidence.

Beginning of Life: Beliefs and Practices

Because life begins at conception, an induced abortion is viewed as murder. If a mother's life is in jeopardy because of the birthing of an infant, it is up to the individual concerned to decide whether to abort. Likewise, JWs avoid contraceptive methods that are abortive, such as intrauterine devices and sterilization. Donor fertilization and surrogacy are condemned.

End of Life: Beliefs and Practices

JWs believe death is akin to sleep. The Bible promises a resurrection of the deceased who are in God's memory ("God's memorial tombs"). The righteous who die look forward to a resurrection, a final judgment, and God's everlasting Kingdom. The resurrected who did not know God will have a chance to learn his ways. Resurrected ones who are judged as wicked go to a quick, permanent death in the grave. Thus:

- JWs do not find comfort in imagining the deceased existing in some kind of afterlife or in being told that God "took" the deceased or decided it was "his time." Instead, they find it comforting to know that the dead "know not anything" and are at rest.

JWs have no distinctive death or burial practices. Cremation is acceptable. Some may resist autopsy for personal reasons but submit to legal authority if it is needed. Active euthanasia or assisting with suicide is forbidden; however, there is no need to employ life-sustaining measures and prolong the dying process. As with all life choices, anything that is not in conflict with Bible teaching is acceptable.

Diet and Lifestyle: Prescriptions and Proscriptions

- No special meats or diets are prescribed. (JWs abstain from meat from which the blood has not been properly drained. Traces of blood in one's meat are acceptable.)

- Alcohol in moderation is acceptable, if it does not reach the point of excess and drunkenness.
- Tobacco and drug abuse are forbidden.
- Sexual relations are only with the marriage partner.
- Cleanliness is highly valued.
- Cultural customs that have false religious meanings (e.g., a cross, Halloween) are avoided.

Additional Miscellaneous Nursing Implications

- JWs do not object to vaccines in general. Acceptance of vaccines that contain minor blood fractions are a matter of personal choice.
- JWs will not want a visit from a chaplain or clergy from another faith tradition. Inquire if they want a visit from a member of their congregation. Treat the lay JW elders as clergy, as they function in that role.
- Patient Visitation Group members from the local congregation can also be called on to provide spiritual and social assistance to members. (Depending on your organization's protocol, the chaplaincy department may initiate any contacts.)
- Hospital Liaison Committees are typically available in large urban communities. They can provide information to JW patients as well as the clinicians and facilitate communication. If providing care for a JW in a rural location and questions regarding treatment arise, contact the JW headquarters' Department of Hospital Information Services (see the earlier section "Illness and Healing").

Ways and Words to Comfort

- Encourage JWs to draw comfort and hope from their faith in the Bible's promises, perhaps asking them if they have a favorite scripture that strengthens them.
- Assure them that while we all handle pain and suffering differently, it is wise to seek help and support from those who love them.
- Invite the bereaved to talk about their loved one, describing his or her life, faith, accomplishments, and hope. Assure the bereaved that grieving is a natural process.

Bibliography

DuBose, E. R., & Penton, M. J. (2002). *The Jehovah's Witness tradition: Religious beliefs and healthcare decisions*. Chicago, IL: The Park Ridge Center. Retrieved from https://www.advocatehealth.com/assets/documents/faith/jehovah5.pdf

Metropolitan Chicago Healthcare Council. (2001). *Guidelines for healthcare providers interacting with Jehovah's Witnesses and their families.* Retrieved from https://www.advocatehealth.com/assets/documents/faith/cgjehovahs_witnesses.pdf

Taylor, E. J. (2012). Jehovah's Witnesses. In E. J. Taylor (Ed.), *Religion: A clinical guide for nursing* (pp. 163–170). New York, NY: Springer Publishing.

Watch Tower Bible & Tract Society of Pennsylvania. (n.d.). *Frequently asked questions about Jehovah's Witnesses.* Retrieved from https://www.jw.org/en/jehovahs-witnesses/faq

10

Christianity: Latter-day Saint

Other Names and Similar Religious Traditions

Several very small denominations have broken off from **the Church of Jesus Christ of Latter-day Saints**. These include the **Community of Christ**. Although Latter-day Saints are often called Mormons or LDS, they prefer to use their full name.

Social and Historical Background

Founded on the teachings of Prophet Joseph Smith, the Latter-day Saint church was organized in 1830 in the northeastern United States. Subsequent persecutions prompted Latter-day Saint migration to the Western Intermountain region. Latter-day Saint churches (i.e., wards) are run by laypersons, including elders (spiritual leaders), ministering visitors (elders who visit members monthly), and bishops (laypersons who preside over the wards). Young adult women and men often serve 18- and 24-month mission stints, respectively.

Joseph Smith understood that Christ's original church was corrupted and disappeared; God's leading and visions for Smith allowed him to restore to earth this truest form of Christianity—Latter-day Saints. Latter-day Saints believe in a personal God, the incarnated Jesus Christ, and the Holy Ghost (given when one joins the church). Latter-day Saints accept that salvation is conferred by the atoning death of Christ and obedience to this gospel. While Latter-day Saints espouse Christian teachings (including baptism by immersion), they have additional unique beliefs. These include promise of eternal life for those who covenant with God (during temple "endowment" rituals); dynamic revelation (whereby God may reveal new understandings through the contemporary prophets and Latter-day Saint leaders); the kingdom of God (Zion) will be in America—a continent Christ visited after his resurrection; temple marriages beget marriages for eternity, and resulting "celestial families" will be blessed to remain together forever in heaven; and endowed members may baptize by proxy unsaved deceased family members.

Worship and Devotional Practices

Latter-day Saints believe in a personal God who can be communicated with during prayer. Latter-day Saints' prayer is typically conversational, allowing for praise and supplication to God as well as quiet listening. Latter-day Saints also encounter God through sacred scriptures, which include not only the King James Version of the Holy Bible but also stories and instruction translated by or revealed to Joseph Smith (i.e., *The Book of Mormon: Another Testament of Jesus Christ*, *The Pearl of Great Price*, *Doctrine and Covenants*). *The Book of Mormon* is considered a second testament of Jesus Christ. Thus, Latter-day Saints are encouraged to study daily the *Bible* and *The Book of Mormon*. Thus:

■ Accommodate and protect devotional time for the Latter-day Saint (e.g., negotiate when and put signage on the patient's door).
■ Latter-day Saint magazines, videos, and religious teaching resources for persons of all ages are available at the church's website (www.lds.org).

Latter-day Saints attend ward services every Sunday; these services include a worship with the sacrament of the Lord's Supper, study, and fellowship. Given it is observed as the Sabbath, Latter-day Saints avoid work, shopping, and secular recreational activities on Sundays. Though not obligated, Latter-day Saints may fast on occasion or for a 24-hour period prior to services on the first Sunday of each month. Thus:

■ Appreciate how spiritually and socially important attending ward services may be to a patient unable to go. Support ways the patient can stay engaged (e.g., receiving ward visitors, watching live-streamed meetings).
■ Audio and video Latter-day Saint and Christian stories for adults and children are available on the Mormon Channel (www.mormonchannel.org). The Latter-day Saint flagship university's television station, BYUtv, also offers inspirational shows and live television.
■ Patients desiring to fast can adjust the fast to their circumstances (e.g., fast from certain foods/drink, fast for only 6 hours, fast from television or cell phone), remembering the purpose of the fast is prayer and faith development, not fasting for its own sake.

- If a patient is unable to attend services and would appreciate receiving the Lord's Supper, facilitate a request to the local bishop or branch president.

Illness and Healing: Beliefs and Practices

Latter-day Saints believe that the body is a temple of God. Thus, humans comprise both a physical and a spiritual being. Given this, Latter-day Saints give effort to living healthfully and benefiting from scientifically based healthcare. Specific health-related guidance is offered in the "Word of Wisdom" (a section in the *Doctrine and Covenants*; see "Diet and Lifestyle"). Illness, tragedy, and suffering are explained by the positive or negative consequences of free will and nature. Because God grants humans the freedom to make choices, health-related consequences result from one's choices or from those around them. Likewise, the laws of nature—even though designed by God—may manifest in ways that cause suffering because of human choices. Regardless of cause, illness and disability allow the believer to spiritually develop and prepare for the next life. Thus:

- Latter-day Saints may consult church policies or spiritual leaders in their faith community when making major health-related decisions. Respect this process.
- Given the emphasis on free choice in determining circumstances as well as the earthly life purpose to become more perfect and godlike, Latter-day Saints may be prone to shame, depression, or other mental health challenges if they perceive themselves to not be measuring up (Lyon, 2013). Although church leaders have counseled members to seek professional help, a Latter-day Saint might worry that seeking mental healthcare is an indicator of faithlessness.
- A sick Latter-day Saint member may request a "priesthood blessing." This healing ritual involves one or two ward elders anointing the patient's head with consecrated olive oil, praying, and pronouncing a healing blessing. Support as necessary (e.g., prepare the patient to receive these visitors, plan care so there are no interruptions).

Beginning of Life: Beliefs and Practices

Latter-day Saints view birth as the entrance of a spirit child into this earthly life (so that the spirit can attain more godlikeness). Thus, Latter-day Saint women are encouraged to marry a Latter-day Saint man and have children. If married in the temple, this celestial marriage is believed to last eternally. In the United States, Latter-day Saint women on average have more children than non–Latter-day Saints. Thus:

- Because of these beliefs about the sanctity of marriage and life, the following stances regarding perinatal decisions are common: contraception is used to space when children are birthed; sterilization is strongly discouraged unless it is necessary; reproductive technologies are acceptable as long as the genes of both parents are used and applied within a context of marriage; surrogacy is discouraged; abortion is immoral unless, after prayer and consultation with spiritual leaders, it is determined to be God's will (e.g., if a mother's life is in jeopardy, the pregnancy resulted from rape or incest, or there is a severe fetal defect).
- Women in unhappy celestial marriages may be especially despairing, given their belief about it lasting not only in this life but also in the next (Lyon, 2013). Consider with the patient a referral to a Latter-day Saint therapist.

End of Life: Beliefs and Practices

As in a play, Latter-day Saints believe that the human spirit proceeds through three acts. First, it exists as a spirit child of God. Then it is born into an earthly body; after the earthly death, the spirit enters a spirit world where it temporarily rests in peace. Then there will be a literal resurrection when the body and spirit are reunited in a perfect form. Earthly life allows one to become more perfect and godlike. The unrighteous will face God's wrath after death. In the spirit world and after the resurrection, celestial families will continue to relate as families in the presence of the Heavenly Father.

Decisions about end-of-life care will reflect these beliefs (e.g., there is no need to prolong earthly life). Strong respect for the laws of the land and the value of life also dictate choices. Assisted suicide and euthanasia are considered murder. Organ donation and autopsies are acceptable. When making major decisions about end-of-life care, Latter-day Saints may consult their spiritual community.

- There are no prescribed rituals for the end of life.
- When the body of an initiated Latter-day Saint is prepared for burial or cremation, ward members may prepare the body by dressing it in the person's temple garments.
- Given beliefs about the next life, comforting words for those who mourn can acknowledge the hope of the resurrection and eternal life as well as recognition of reunion with family and friends.

Diet and Lifestyle: Prescriptions and Proscriptions

A literature review concluded that due to lifestyle proscriptions, Latter-day Saints in the Western Intermountain region experience greater physical well-being than their non–Latter-day Saint counterparts (de Diego Cordero & Badanta Romero, 2017). Latter-day Saints abstain from all forms of tobacco, alcohol, and addictive drugs (unless a physician prescribes them). Latter-day Saints also do not consume coffee or caffeinated tea. Although not proscribed, meat may be eaten with moderation. Grains, fruits, and vegetables are encouraged. Thus:

- Assess drink and dietary preferences, if needed.

Latter-day Saints' lifestyle promotes family cohesion and conservative sexual mores. One evening per week (usually Monday), families take time to pray, study Latter-day Saint teachings, and play together; they may also have a shorter family worship time every day. Extramarital sex, pornography, masturbation, and homosexuality are proscribed, as is passionate physical intimacy between a dating couple. Members are encouraged to dress modestly. Thus:

- When addressing issues of sexuality with Latter-day Saint patients for whom it has been altered (e.g., hemiplegics), discuss sexual practices that are aligned with Latter-day Saint laws of chastity.

Additional Miscellaneous Nursing Implications

Latter-day Saints have a strong system for supporting their own. If a member becomes ill, it is likely that the system will soon identify the need and implement action to provide support. That is, a member is automatically seen once every month by men and women of the church during ministering visits. These lay leaders will directly aid or organize support. Even for Latter-day Saints who are hospitalized away from home, the local bishop can arrange for his ward members to provide support. Thus:

- Facilitate connection with this source of support for patients if it is needed and desired, by making a request to the chaplain or directly to the nearest ward's bishop.

Endowed (initiated Latter-day Saints who have a made a solemn vow to live uprightly) may wear "temple garments." These undergarments are reminders of their sacred covenant and are considered symbols of protection. Thus:

- Handle these undergarments with respect; when they do not interfere with procedures, allow the patient to wear them.

Ways and Words to Comfort

■ Visit Disability Resources on the Latter-day Saint church's website. On the Adversity page (www.lds.org/topics/disability/scriptures/quotes/adversity?lang=eng&old=true) are numerous inspirational quotes from Latter-day Saint spiritual leaders. For example:

> No pain that we suffer, no trial that we experience is wasted. It ministers to our education, to the development of such qualities as patience, faith, fortitude and humility. All that we suffer and all that we endure, especially when we endure it patiently, builds up our characters, purifies our hearts, expands our souls, and makes us more tender and charitable, more worthy to be called the children of God. (O. F. Whitney, as cited in The Church of Jesus Christ of Latter-day Saints, n.d., para. 6)

Bibliography

Abbott, D. (Ed.). (2002). *The Latter-day Saints tradition: Religious beliefs and healthcare decisions*. Chicago, IL: The Park Ridge Center. Retrieved from https://www.advocatehealth.com/assets/documents/faith/latter-day_saints_tradition.pdf

The Church of Jesus Christ of Latter-day Saints. (n.d.). *Adversity*. Retrieved from https://www.lds.org/topics/disability/scriptures/quotes/adversity?lang=eng&old=true

de Diego Cordero, R., & Badanta Romero, B. (2017). Health impacts of religious practices and beliefs associated with The Church of Jesus Christ of Latter-day Saints. *Journal of Religion & Health, 56*(4), 1371–1380. doi:10.1007/s10943-016-0348-y

Lyon, S. J. (2013). Psychotherapy and the Mormon faith. *Journal of Religion & Health, 52*(2), 622–630. doi:10.1007/s10943-013-9677-2

Mormon.org. (n.d.). *Articles of faith*. Retrieved from https://www.mormon.org/beliefs/articles-of-faith

Top, B. L., & Top, J. B. (2012). Latter-day Saints (Mormons). In E. J. Taylor (Ed.), *Religion: A clinical guide for nurses* (pp. 181–190). New York, NY: Springer Publishing.

11

Christianity: Lutheran

Other Names and Similar Religious Traditions

In the United States, the largest denomination of Lutherans is the **Evangelical Lutheran Church in America** (ELCA). There are, however, several other American Lutheran denominations (e.g., **Lutheran Church—Missouri Synod**, the next largest) as well as numerous other Evangelical Lutheran churches organized in countries worldwide.

Social and Historical Background

Lutheranism originated with Martin Luther (1483–1546), a German Catholic monk whose attempts to reform the church led to the Protestant Reformation. What distinguished Luther's beliefs was that people are saved by grace through faith in Jesus Christ, not by their works or effort to achieve it. Immigrants brought Lutheranism to North America in the 1800s. The different Lutheran denominations were originally explained by geographic or immigrant cultures; however, in 1988, when three main Lutheran denominations joined, those that did not join did so for doctrinal differences explained by more conservative interpretations of the Bible. Thus:

- Non-ELCA Lutherans will likely hold more conservative views and lifestyles (e.g., regarding abortion, homosexuality, and ordination of women).

Worship and Devotional Practices

See Chapter 21. The *Lutheran Book of Prayer* (Kinnaman, 2005) contains morning and evening prayers for each day of the week; these are designed to be prayed by an individual.

Illness and Healing: Beliefs and Practices

These practices do not differ substantially from those of other mainline Christians (see Chapter 21).

Beginning of Life: Beliefs and Practices

While ELCA Lutherans believe abortion should be a "last resort" taken before a fetus' life can be sustained outside the womb, Missouri Synod Lutherans take a more conservative stance and believe abortion is a sin and should never be performed unless it is to save the life of the mother (Lutheran Church—Missouri Synod, n.d.). ELCA recognizes and accepts the tension of diverse biblically based views regarding same-sex marriages, whereas more conservative Lutherans believe them to be sinful. Thus:

- When pertinent, assessment regarding what a patient believes about abortion will be helpful.
- Referral to online ELCA statement of belief in this regard may alleviate guilt for a woman who has had an abortion.

End of Life: Beliefs and Practices

- Organ transplantation is encouraged.
- Cremation is acceptable.
- A service of Commendation for the Dying performed by a pastor is encouraged. This service allows for prayer just prior to death.

Diet and Lifestyle: Prescriptions and Proscriptions

These practices are similar to those of other mainline Christians (see Chapter 21).

Additional Miscellaneous Nursing Implications

See Chapter 21.

Ways and Words to Comfort

The *Evangelical Lutheran Worship, Pastoral Care* book contains numerous prayers and scriptural reading suggestions for many different life needs or events, including health and healing (Chapter 5) and death (Chapter 6). Chapter 8.4 contains prayers and readings for a long list of circumstances (e.g., anxiety, fear, guilt, loneliness, anger, gratitude, disability, childbirth). Although this book is available for purchase, the preliminary draft is available for free online

(Evangelical Lutheran Church of America, 2007). Prayers in this book include:

- For physical illness: "O God, the strength of the weak and the comfort of sufferers: Mercifully hear our prayers and grant to your servant [patient name] the help of your power, that *her/his* sickness may be turned into health and our anxiety into joy; through Jesus Christ our Lord. (5.2.2.1.)" (p. 39)
- For emotional distress: "Merciful God, you give us the grace that helps in time of need. Surround [patient name] with your steadfast love and lighten *her/his* burden. By the power of your Spirit, free *her/him* from distress and give *her/him* a new mind and heart made whole in the name of the risen Christ. (5.2.21.1.)" (p. 47)

Bibliography

Association of Religion Data Archives. (n.d.). *Lutheran family. Christian. Religion family trees.* Retrieved from http://www.thearda.com/denoms/Families/trees/familytree_lutheran.asp

Evangelical Lutheran Church of America. (2007). *Evangelical Lutheran worship pastoral care: Readings, prayers, and occasional services (Provisional draft for review).* Retrieved from http://parksidelutheran.org/ELW PastoralCare_ProvisionalReview_200710.pdf

Evangelical Lutheran Church in America. (2018). *Faith.* Retrieved from https://www.elca.org/Faith

Kinnaman, S. A. (Ed.). (2005). *Lutheran book of prayer* (5th ed.). St. Louis, MO: Concordia.

Luoma, J., & Sundberg, W. (2012). *Lutherans.* In E. J. Taylor (Ed.), *Religion: A clinical guide for nurses* (pp. 191–196). New York, NY: Springer Publishing.

Lutheran Church—Missouri Synod. (n.d.). *Belief and practice.* Retrieved from https://www.lcms.org/about/beliefs

12

Christianity: Methodist, Moravian, Wesleyan, and Holiness Denominations

Other Names and Similar Religious Traditions

A Methodist denomination or church name will likely include the words or phrases Methodist Church, United Methodist, Evangelical Methodist, or Free Methodist. Similar denominations include **Moravian**, **Wesleyan**, and those from **Holiness** traditions (e.g., Church of the Nazarene, Salvation Army, and Church of God [Anderson, IN]) and African American Methodist Episcopal denominations (see Chapter 8).

Social and Historical Background

The 18th-century English brothers John (an Anglican priest) and Charles (a prolific hymnist) Wesley led the movement that later evolved to become Methodism. They were influenced by the post-Protestant Reformation pietistic Christians (now known as Moravians or Unity Brethren) who emphasized the importance of personal piety—of personal spiritual experience and relationship with God. Methodism emphasized not only personal piety but also social change. Thus, subsequent iterations of Methodism (i.e., Wesleyanism and Holiness denominations) also strive to transform and bring healing to individuals and societies.

Worship and Devotional Practices

Given the emphasis on Bible study and devotion to God, Methodists, Wesleyans, Pietists, and Holiness Christians often spend a dedicated time each day for personal devotion or worship, reading the Bible and/or Christian inspiration and prayer. To seek God, Methodists use the quadrilateral of scripture (the Bible), religious tradition, reason, and personal experience. Thus:

- Provide uninterrupted time and, if need be, Christian literature. Denominational websites provide daily devotions that are short and easily read to the patient if needed.
  - Prayers and faith stories are available on the United Methodist Church (UMC) website (www.umc.org/topics/topic-prayers-and-meditations), as are daily devotionals (www.upperroom.org/devotionals).
  - Daily devotionals are available on the Wesleyan Church website (www.wesleyan.org/category/devotions).

For Methodists, there are two sacraments: Communion (or Lord's Supper), which is served at church services once per month or weekly, and a water baptism for children as soon as possible if there is a parent or sponsor willing to provide the child with religious nurture. (Communion "wine" is grape juice, likely served from a communal cup.) In contrast, members of the Salvation Army do not view communion or baptism as necessary. Whereas some will baptize by immersing or sprinkling water on part of the body, Church of God (Anderson, IN) baptisms involve total immersion. Thus:

- If a baby is terminally ill, Methodist parents would want to have their baby baptized. Methodists do not, however, believe that a baby will not go to heaven if the child is not baptized. Given only clergy perform baptisms, a referral to a chaplain should be made at such time if possible.

Illness and Healing: Beliefs and Practices

Beliefs and practices regarding illness and healing are similar to those of other mainline Christians. Healing services (with laying on of hands, anointing the forehead with oil, receiving communion, and reading a Bible passage) are not intended as curative but as creating an atmosphere where one's relationship with God is nourished—which is healing.

Beginning of Life: Beliefs and Practices

Beliefs and practices regarding beginning of life are similar to those of other mainline Protestants (see Chapter 21).

End of Life: Beliefs and Practices

Most end-of-life perspectives are similar to those of other mainline Protestants (see Chapter 21). Methodists believe that after death there is both an intermediate state while one awaits the Resurrection Day and an immediate being with God; however, this belief varies greatly between members.

Diet and Lifestyle: Prescriptions and Proscriptions

Care for one's body as the temple of God may be interpreted more conservatively among persons in these traditions than among those in some other mainstream Christian denominations. For example, whereas the Wesleyan Church expects members to abstain from alcohol, United Methodists advise judicious consumption. Indeed, Wesleyans also oppose use of tobacco and harmful drugs, unless they are for medicinal purposes. These denominations often promote a healthful lifestyle within congregational venues. Thus:

■ The body as a "temple of God" may be an appropriate motivation for health promotion.

Additional Miscellaneous Nursing Implications

■ United Methodist churches sometimes have a faith community nurse or Steven Ministers (laypersons trained to visit the sick, the bereaved, or those experiencing a substantial challenge—in or out of the church); these persons are a resource for community-based support.

Ways and Words to Comfort

See Chapter 21.

■ A UMC prayer about turning to God during times of trouble is available at www.umc.org/what-we-believe/a-united-methodist -prayer-turning-to-god-in-days-of-trouble. An adaptation of this prayer reads: "Dear Lord, When all we can do is cry; when loneliness seems overwhelming, when there is death and destruction . . . be present to us. May we be untiring in living with your grace and love. Amen."

Bibliography

Church of the Nazarene. (n.d.). *Nazarene in a glance*. Retrieved from http://nazarene.org/nazarene-glance

Free Methodist Church. (n.d.). *Home*. Retrieved from http://fmcusa.org/uniquelyfm

Simonds, B. (2012). Methodists (Wesleyans). In E. J. Taylor (Ed.), *Religion: A clinical guide for nurses* (pp. 197–204). New York, NY: Springer Publishing.

Unitas Fratrum. (n.d.). *The origin and growth*. Retrieved from http://www.unitasfratrum.org/index.php/origin-growth-of-the-unitas-fratrum

United Methodist Church. (n.d.). *United Methodist communications*. Retrieved from http://www.umc.org/who-we-are/united-methodist-communications

Wesleyan Church. (2016). *Church and culture*. Indianapolis, IN: Wesleyan Publishing House. Retrieved from https://www.wesleyan.org/church-and-culture-booklet-246

13

Christianity: Metropolitan Community Church

Other Names and Similar Religious Traditions

Officially, this Christian denomination is the Universal Fellowship of Metropolitan Community Churches (MCC, 2013).

Social and Historical Background

The first MCC worship service occurred in 1968 in the living room of a former Pentecostal minister who had been defrocked because of his homosexual orientation. Whereas this Christian denomination provides a home for lesbian/gay/bisexual/transgender/queer (LGBTQ) persons, it is purposefully accepting of diverse people and of diverse theologies. MCC core values include inclusion, community, spiritual transformation, and justice. The desire for social justice leads MCC to work toward the protection of human and civil rights, including LGBTQ equality (e.g., same-sex marriage).

Worship and Devotional Practices

Given the diverse Christian backgrounds of its members, MCC's Sunday worship services and personal devotional practices vary (see Chapter 21).

Illness and Healing: Beliefs and Practices

See Chapter 21. Most Christian (as well as Islamic) church teachings consider homosexual behavior as sinful. Thus, MCC LGBTQ members likely have had or continue to spiritually struggle to respect their personhood. This may contribute to the higher prevalence of mental health challenges among LGBTQ members.

Beginning of Life: Beliefs and Practices

See Chapter 21.

End of Life: Beliefs and Practices

Given a history that includes the AIDS epidemic, LGBT communities are typically extraordinarily supportive of those in their midst who are dying (see also Chapter 21).

Diet and Lifestyle: Prescriptions and Proscriptions

See Chapter 21.

Additional Miscellaneous Nursing Implications

Like mid-20th-century psychiatrists, many Christian (and non-Christian) faith traditions historically adopted the position that being LGBTQ was an aberration. Among Christians, homosexuality was believed to be sinful, given several biblical texts describing deviant sexual practices as immoral. Although lagging behind the trend in secular society, Christians are increasingly affirming and inclusive of LGBTQs. Denominations that endorse nearly literal interpretations of the Bible, however, position themselves today as "loving the sinner, but not the sin of homosexuality." Thus:

- Appreciate LGBTQ Christians may have "baggage" about the church they grew up in yet yearn for religious fellowship. Listen deeply and respond with empathy. Outgrowing childhood images of God will allow spiritual and psychological well-being (e.g., God as love vs. God as a bearded, old man).
- Provide nonjudgmental and respectful support. Remember that spiritual care does not entail attempting to convince a patient to adopt certain beliefs or behaviors. Furthermore, the Christian nurse will do well to remember that conversion is the work of God, not the nurse.
- See Chapter 21.

Ways and Words to Comfort

- The MCC website (www.mcchurch.org/resources/mcc -theologies) contains a "Theological Resources" page with links to several documents that will help the Christian LGBTQ person read the Bible with "new eyes" (e.g., "Coming Out as Sacrament").

- MCC founder, Troy Perry, and recent leader Dr. Nancy Wilson have published several books for Christian LGBTs (available from most book retailers) that can help Christian LGBT patients embrace their sexual identity.

Bibliography

McDonald, K. (2018). Social support and mental health in LGBTQ adolescents: A review of the literature. *Issues in Mental Health Nursing, 39*(1), 16–29. doi:10.1080/01612840.2017.1398283

Metropolitan Community Churches. (n.d.). *Overview*. Retrieved from https://www.mccchurch.org/overview

Paul, J. (2017). The varieties of religious responses to homosexuality: A content and tonal analysis of articles in *Pastoral Psychology* from 1950 to 2015 regarding sexual minorities. *Pastoral Psychology, 66*(1), 79–101. doi:10.1007/s11089-016-0717-1

Valentine, S. E., & Shepherd, J. C. (2018). A systematic review of social stress and mental health among transgender and gender non-conforming people in the United States. *Clinical Psychology Review, 66*, 24–38. doi:10.1016/j.cpr.2018.03.003

14

Christianity: Orthodox

Other Names and Similar Religious Traditions

Orthodox Christianity is composed of patriarchates that are generally organized along national boundaries (e.g., Serbia, Russia, Romania, Japan, Finland) and will have the term Orthodox in their name. These churches can be categorized as **Oriental** (comprising primarily churches in northeastern Africa and the Middle East) and **Eastern** (including patriarchates primarily from eastern Europe). Some Orthodox Christians are organized in the United States under the **Orthodox Church of America**.

Social and Historical Background

Orthodox Christians (OCs) believe their religion is the original organized Christian tradition. During much of the first millennium CE, the Christian church was organized into five geographic areas, with centers (patriarchates) located in Rome, Constantinople, Alexandria, Antioch, and Jerusalem. In 1054, after mounting political and theological tensions between the western patriarchate of Rome and the others, the Christian church split. The Roman patriarchate became the Roman Catholic church, whereas the remaining patriarchates remained united as OCs. (Thus, OCs are neither Catholic nor Protestant.) OCs have been active evangelists, explaining why OC can be found around the world and why in North America an OC congregation can include ethnically diverse members. The honored leader of OC is the Patriarch of Constantinople; however, he is viewed as "first among equals."

Worship and Devotional Practices

OC communal worship in a church is the Divine Liturgy, held every Sunday, on feast days, and on special occasions. Thus:

- Because OCs place emphasis on faith within the context of community, those who are unable to attend Divine Liturgy or other church events may be at risk for spiritual distress. Many OC churches livestream their Divine Liturgies. This allows patients who cannot attend on Sundays or feast days to "attend."
- OCs fast prior to Divine Liturgies so as to empty oneself of food and be ready to receive Christ during Holy Communion. A rule of thumb is that one is to fast the number of hours that is one's age— up to 8 to 12 hours (e.g., a 1-year-old fasts for 1 hour, whereas an adult will begin the fast Saturday night). Although the sick and elderly who need to eat more frequently are exempt, they may need encouragement that "God [or the priest] understands."

The OC follows a liturgical calendar that specifies 12 Great Feast Days as well as Pascha (Easter). Likewise, the 40 days prior to Pascha and Holy Week as well as the 40 days prior to Christmas (celebrated by some on December 25 and some on January 7) are Lenten seasons for observing ascetic practices that strengthen self-discipline and faith. Fasting is practiced not only during these Lents but also on some feast days and some Wednesdays and Fridays. Thus:

- Fasting involves, at minimum, not eating meat; ideally, it involves fasting from dairy products, eggs, oil, and fish. Permissible foods include any fruit or vegetables, nuts, grains, honey, and margarine. More fundamental, however, is observing moderation in what is eaten or drunk. The seriously ill and hospitalized are exempt from the Wednesday and Friday fasts but may prefer to still observe them. Given the complexity of fasting observances and variation in how they are practiced, ask OC patients what they wish to eat daily.
- Feast days are typically celebrated not only with prayers and special rituals but also with family and food. These will vary depending on the family's culture. Encourage family to observe these celebrations, even if in a modified way, with patients who are hospitalized (e.g., bringing food).

OCs also worship privately when they read the Bible, pray and meditate, or act with compassion. Thus:

- If a patient wants someone to read scripture, know that the New Testament books of Matthew, Mark, Luke, and John (the Gospels) that describe the life of Jesus may be most appreciated, while

Epistles (letters written by apostles after Jesus's time) and Psalms are other top selections (see the appendix). The patient may prefer a selection from the liturgical calendar, the schedule specifying Bible readings for each day of the year (see oca.org/readings).

■ If obtaining a copy of a Bible for an OC, know that the Orthodox Study Bible and New King James Version are preferred.

■ Although some OCs may not wish to pray with a person of a different faith, they may appreciate a read prayer from the *Ancient Faith Prayer Book* or from the Orthodox Church of America's *Prayers for Orthodox Christians* (available online at oca.org/orthodoxy/prayers). In general, OCs prefer a read prayer rather than a colloquial prayer.

Illness and Healing: Beliefs and Practices

See Chapter 21. OCs place emphasis on finding meaning for suffering in the modeling of Jesus and saints who likewise suffered. Ethical health-related decisions are to be guided by the Bible and church teachings, yet ultimately it is up to the believer (in the context of their relationships) to discern. The discernment process will likely be guided by the local priest or a spiritual father (a spiritual mentor someone may consult one or two times per year throughout life).

When devout OCs become ill, they often make sure to have the local parish priest informed. OCs may request the sacraments of Holy Confession and Holy Communion, as these are believed to heal "soul and body." Although some may misunderstand the Sacrament of Holy Unction as appropriate only at the end of life, it is an anointing service that may be received for *any* health challenge. Thus:

■ When there is a substantial change in health, determine if the patient wishes for OC clergy contact. If it is not the role of the organization's chaplain to contact the local OC parish, facilitate this process (e.g., ask the family to make the contact or call the parish office). OC rituals (including communion) cannot be administered by non-OC clergy; indeed, OC patients may be hesitant of any religious support from non-OCs.

Beginning of Life: Beliefs and Practices

Perinatal practices reflect not only value for the sanctity and dignity of human life (having been made in the image of God) but also the procreative (rather than hedonistic) purpose of marriage. Given such values, abortion is not practiced (unless the mother's life is in jeopardy and those involved are consulted), neither is sex selection, fertilization by a donor, sterilization, or contraception involving postconception abortion (e.g., intrauterine device [IUD] or "morning-after pill").

Several religious "rites of initiation" are practiced after a birth, including those that involve naming the infant, baptism, chrismation (welcoming/sealing of the Holy Spirit), and welcoming the mother and child back to church (40 days after birth). Whereas these will only be performed by the OC priest or parish clergy at the behest of the family, the baptism may be done in an emergency if the infant's death is imminent and no clergy are available. Stillborn babies are not baptized. Thus:

- Baptism, a sacrament that signifies the spiritual birth into Christ, should be performed by the OC clergy. When a death is expected, proactively contact the family's OC priest immediately. In case of a dire emergency when OC clergy or other clergy are unable to be present, a nurse can inquire if the parents wish for a Christian nurse to baptize the infant. If yes, then proceed as follows: (1) Obtain a deep basin with clean water. (2) Speak the following: "The servant of God, [say the name of infant] is baptized in the name of the Father, Son, and Holy Spirit. Amen." (3) After naming each member of the Godhead, submerge the infant.

End of Life: Beliefs and Practices

At death, the soul leaves the physical body. There is a reunion of soul with the body during the resurrection occurring at the Second Coming of Christ. Although there is a Partial Judgment at death, after the Second Coming, there will be a Full Judgment, when whether one receives eternal communion (heaven) or separation from God (hell) will be decided. OC Liturgy prayers include reminders that one is always to prepare for one's death. Practices surrounding the end of life reflect the hope of the resurrection as well as a strong belief that, even after death, one's body remains "the tabernacle of the Holy Spirit." Thus:

- When death or loss of consciousness becomes imminent, facilitate the OC's priest's celebration of Holy Unction or the "Service for the Parting of the Soul From the Body" (e.g., create space, avoid interruptions). The patient needs to be conscious for this rite; thereafter, pain management that counters awareness can be implemented.
- There are other death-related religio-cultural practices. These, however, vary by tradition and culture. Given the complexity of these practices and the naiveté of many OCs regarding these practices, it is essential to involve the local priest. Anticipate these needs if the patient and family so desire.

- Once the patient has died, continue to very respectfully treat the body as "the tabernacle of the Holy Spirit." Thus, bodies may be embalmed but are not to be cremated or submitted to an unnecessary autopsy. Many do not donate their organs. Even when the body becomes an organ donor or cadaver, it must be treated with dignity. Indeed, organ donation is acceptable as long as burial rituals can be practiced.
- The family may request a priest to pray before the deceased body is moved.
- Extraordinary interventions to prolong life or hasten death (e.g., assisted suicide, active euthanasia) are not to be implemented.

Bereavement practices involve several specific times for prayers and liturgies. These include several times during the first 40 days after death, at 6 months, and annual anniversaries of death.

Diet and Lifestyle: Prescriptions and Proscriptions

See the earlier section "Worship and Devotional Practices" regarding fasting. OCs pray both before and after a meal to show their gratitude to God (see Chapter 21).

Additional Miscellaneous Nursing Implications

- Religious support should be provided by an OC priest, parish nurse/faith community nurse, or trained lay minister; non-OC spiritual carers cannot be substituted. OC clergy are always eager to provide pastoral care to OC parishioners.

Ways and Words to Comfort

- To comfort the bereaved (even years after a death), simply say, "Memory eternal." This phrase reminds them that their loved one is in heaven eternally.
- "And we know that all things work together for good to them that love God" (Romans 8:28).
- An OC prayer for the sick (oca.org/orthodoxy/prayers/for -the-sick) is as follows: "O Christ, Who alone art our Defender: Visit and heal Thy suffering servant [insert name], delivering him/her from sickness and grievous pains. Raise him/her up that he/she may sing to Thee and praise Thee without ceasing, through the prayers of the Theotokos, O Thou Who along lovest mankind." (Note: *Theotokos* [Mother of God] is Mary, the mother of Jesus.)
- The ancient "Jesus Prayer" is helpful during times of extremis, as it can be prayed repetitively to focus attention: "O Lord Jesus

Christ, Son of God, Have mercy on me, a sinner." (See oca.org/ orthodoxy/prayers/the-jesus-prayer.)

- Icons, experienced as pictures into heaven, provide much comfort. Icons are pictures of Jesus, Mary, or saints and can be palm sized or larger. A patient will likely have a preferred icon. Invite the family to bring an icon to the patient's bedside and place it where it can be viewed by the patient.

- A prayer rope (a cord with knots, the size of a bracelet or larger) or crocheted cross (in the style of the patient's Orthodox tradition) can be placed in the hands of the patient to provide spiritual comfort and guide prayer.

Bibliography

Harakas, S. S. (1999). *The Orthodox Christian tradition: Religious beliefs and healthcare decisions.* Chicago, IL: The Park Ridge Center. Retrieved from https://www.advocatehealth.com/assets/documents/faith/orthodox _christian.pdf

Matusiak, J. (2012). *Orthodox Christians..* In E. J. Taylor (Ed.), *Religion: A clinical guide for nurses* (pp. 221–226). New York, NY: Springer Publishing.

Orthodox Church in America. (n.d.). *The Orthodox faith.* Retrieved from https://oca.org/orthodoxy

World Council of Churches. (n.d.-a). *Orthodox churches (Eastern).* Retrieved from https://www.oikoumene.org/en/church-families/orthodox-churches -eastern

World Council of Churches. (n.d.-b). *Orthodox churches (Oriental).* Retrieved from https://www.oikoumene.org/en/church-families/orthodox-churches -oriental

15

Christianity: Pentecostal

Other Names and Similar Religious Traditions

The Pentecostal family includes over 30 denominations, the largest of which are the **Assemblies of God** and the **Church of God in Christ**. Other denominations include the **Church of God** (Cleveland, TN); **Foursquare Gospel**; **Pentecostal Holiness Church**; **United Pentecostal Church International**; **Vineyard USA; Full Gospel Fellowship;** and **Calvary Chapel**. Pentecostals often describe themselves as belonging to the "Apostolic Faith," "Full Gospel," or "Latter Rain." The **Church of God in Christ**, **Pentecostal Assemblies of the World**, and other Pentecostal denominations that are primarily African American can be better understood by also reading Chapter 8.

Social and Historical Background

Pentecostalism, an outgrowth of the Holiness movement (which was an outgrowth of Methodism), has its roots in the early 1900s in the United States. The term Pentecostal derives from the initial event of Pentecost, when the earliest Christians received an outpouring ("baptizing") of the Holy Spirit (the "Comforter" or Spirit that is the gift and empowering presence of God in humans). For some Pentecostals, this baptism of the Holy Spirit is evidenced when one "speaks in tongues" (also called "prayer language" or "praying in the Spirit"). All, however, are to live with openness to the work of the Holy Spirit through "signs and wonders," or supernatural gifts or miracles.

Because of Pentecostals' emphasis on the Second Coming, they are eager to talk about their personal faith and evangelize. Pentecostals are also eager to be "saved" (invite Jesus into their lives) and experience sanctification by the Word, Water, and Spirit; however, some denominations differ regarding whether this is a one-time event or a lifetime process. Likewise, while many Pentecostal Holiness denominations accept a Trinitarian doctrine (i.e., that the facets of God include God as Father, as Holy Spirit, and as Jesus Christ), a few perceive God in a "Oneness modality" and baptize in the name of Jesus. Many "Word Church" believers accept positive confession theology, or the belief that God blesses believers with physical and material as well as spiritual well-being.

Worship and Devotional Practices

Many will read the Bible (the "Word") every day; its content are considered inerrant and infallible. Pentecostals will likely attend Sunday services weekly, where communion is usually served once a month. Religious nurture may also come from watching or listening to religious programming on television or Internet sources or listening to the Bible or other religious books "on tape." (Many televangelists are Pentecostal.) Sources likely to be appreciated include:

- ag.org/Beliefs/Our-Core-Doctrines/Divine-Healing (Assemblies of God website on divine healing where many recordings on the topic exist)
- ag.org/Resources/Devotionals (Assemblies of God website page where links to daily devotionals can be found)
- www.evangelmagazine.com (Church of God [Cleveland, TN] webpage for a devotional magazine)
- iphc.org/discipleship (International Pentecostal Holiness Church webpage with devotionals)
- www.upci.org/resources/magazines (United Pentecostal Church International's webpage where church magazines for adults, youth, and ladies can be read online)

Illness and Healing: Beliefs and Practices

Pentecostals believe in "divine healing." That is, because of the death of Jesus, believers can receive not only forgiveness from sins but also physical healing. Such healing is believed to be a confirmation of the Word that is preached. Thus, it is typical that after the sermon at a Pentecostal service, attendees will be invited to approach the pastor (who is assisted by lay leaders) to receive a prayer for sickness or disability. Thus:

- Whereas most seek traditional Western medical care, there are some who will think that doing so exhibits a lack of faith and will not receive such healthcare.
- Likewise, some charismatic Pentecostals believe that because Jesus took human suffering on himself, there is no need for humans to

experience suffering. Thus, if one suffers or continues to be sick, it reflects a lack of faith or a punishment for a particular sin.

- Most, however, recognize the mystery of suffering and how it allows spiritual transformation.

Pentecostal leaders will also pray at a patient's bedside and perform an anointing if requested (i.e., a drop of oil on the forehead). Thus:

- Appreciate that there may be a group of people who gather for this special prayer service; they may pray in a somewhat loud voice, sing, or speak in tongues, with hands raised.
- The patient may also ask the pastor to pray over an object (e.g., handkerchief) that they can then retain on their body as a reminder of the healing; respect this.

Beginning of Life: Beliefs and Practices

The Assemblies of God and Church of God (Cleveland, TN), given it is a large denomination, provides members with statements to guide moral decision making about a number of topics, including abortion. The Assemblies of God statement regarding abortion and reproductive issues represents well what other Pentecostals espouse. It advises in vitro fertilization and contraception are personal matters requiring prayerfulness (but reminds that intrauterine devices [IUDs] and morning-after pills are abortive); states that abortion is evil and cloning is immoral; and encourages biomedical research, including stem cell research, if it is "reverent and responsible" (Assemblies of God, 2010).

Most Pentecostals believe in a water baptism by immersion when one can make such a decision; they do not baptize infants.

End of Life: Beliefs and Practices

Life, to its very end, is sacred. Therefore, euthanasia and assisted dying are believed immoral, as they devalue life and suffering. After death, there is eternal life for those who are saved (i.e., a literal heaven) and eternal punishment for the wicked (i.e., a literal hell without any ending). When believers die, their bodies await a resurrection that will occur at the Second Coming of Jesus Christ. Thus:

- It is comforting for the dying to remember that they will soon see Jesus and that there will be reunion with loved ones in heaven.
- It is discomforting for family if it is thought that a dying family member is not saved.

There are no specified burial practices.

Chapter 15 Christianity: Pentecostal

Diet and Lifestyle: Prescriptions and Proscriptions

There are no diet recommendations; however, abstinence from all forms of alcohol is expected. Avoidance of ethanol in medications, flavorings, and substances with traces is unnecessary. Gambling is opposed, given its injurious, immoral nature.

Additional Miscellaneous Nursing Implications

- If a patient does speak in tongues, respect that this is his or her way of communing with God; it is not indicative of mental illness or stuttering.
- Pentecostal patients may be more likely to have a vision, dream, or spiritual experience where they encounter a spiritual being (e.g., angel, Jesus, God); allowing patients to talk about such an experience will allow them to make sense of it and find comfort.
- Some churches (or groups of churches) have benevolence ministries that assist needy persons in the community. Some churches will have trained volunteers who visit the sick.
- Patients who wonder if their illness is a punishment are at risk for emotional distress as well as spiritual struggle. If the patient consents, make a referral to an expert chaplain or trained counselor.

Ways and Words to Comfort

- "By His stripes we are healed" (Isaiah 53:5) is commonly cited to affirm divine healing.
- A colloquial prayer, especially one that includes praise, will likely be readily welcomed (see Chapter 21).

Bibliography

Assemblies of God. (2010). *Sanctity of human life: Abortion and reproductive issues.* Retrieved from https://ag.org/Beliefs/Position-Papers/Abortion-Sanctity-of-Human-Life

Assemblies of God. (n.d.). *About.* Retrieved from https://ag.org/About

The Foursquare Church. (n.d.). *About us.* Retrieved from https://www.foursquare.org/about

Full Gospel Ministerial Association of America. (2018). *Tenets of faith.* Retrieved from http://www.fgmaa.org/site/cpage.asp?cpage_id=140015394&sec_id=140005236

IPHC. (2018). *Who we are.* Retrieved from https://iphc.org/about-us

Mathew, T. K. (2012). Pentecostals. In E. J. Taylor (Ed.), *Religion: A clinical guide for nurses* (pp. 227–232). New York, NY: Springer Publishing.

United Pentecostal Church International. (n.d.). *About the UPCI.* Retrieved from https://www.upci.org/about/about-the-upci

16

Christianity: Presbyterian and Other Reformed Denominations

Other Names and Similar Religious Traditions

The World Council of Churches lists about 90 Reformed denominations worldwide. In the United States, 18 Reformed denominations exist (Association of Religion Data Archives [ARDA], 2018). The most common include **Christian Reformed Church in North America** (www.crcna.org), **Reformed Church in America** (www.rca.org), **Presbyterian Church in America** (www.pcaac.org), and **Presbyterian Church** (United States)—by far the largest (www.pcusa.org).

Social and Historical Background

The Reformed family of Christian churches evolved during the Protestant Reformation in Europe during the 1500s. Immigrants from Europe brought the Reformed denominations to North America; this family of denominations has subsequently been introduced by missionaries to Africa, Korea, and countries in the South Pacific. Given this Reformation background, it is easy to understand how key tenets include the following: God is sovereign, His son (Jesus Christ) is the head of the church, salvation is by grace alone through Jesus Christ, and believers are called to act justly to transform the world and to oppose idolatry and tyranny. Although the Bible is the primary authority for the church, these denominations also are guided by several historic Creeds and Confessions. These churches are led collaboratively between lay leaders and clergy. Values embedded in these believers include promoting social justice and human wholeness and education (clergy and laity alike tend to be well educated).

Worship and Devotional Practices

Worship and devotional practices are similar to those of other Christians (see Chapter 21). Communion may be served weekly, but it is often monthly at church. Some follow the liturgical calendar.

Illness and Healing: Beliefs and Practices

See Chapter 21 for common Christian beliefs and practices. No specific practices are prescribed or proscribed in Reformed denominations. Adherents are encouraged to remember their lives are not their own and that they are to be good stewards of life. Thus, they are to pursue health for themselves and for society. Religious leaders can provide an "anointing with oil" along with prayer for those who need healing, and likewise, a "laying on of hands" (on the head or shoulder).

Beginning of Life: Beliefs and Practices

See Chapter 21. No religious beliefs or practices surrounding childbirth are unique to Reformed denominations. Although baptism can occur at any age, it is often performed for infants. If the infant is dying, it is not theologically required or essential to baptize. Baptism, however, may be performed if requested by the parents. There is no religious mandate for male infant circumcision.

End of Life: Beliefs and Practices

These denominations have no religious specifications regarding the preparation of the body, burial over cremation, or the time at which the body must be interred. Adherents believe there will be an afterlife in the presence of God where all will be well.

Diet and Lifestyle: Prescriptions and Proscriptions

There are no specific prescriptions and proscriptions regarding diet and lifestyle, other than those that promote health.

Additional Miscellaneous Nursing Implications

There are no specific nursing implications that are unique for Reformed patients that are not common to other Christian traditions (see Chapter 21).

Ways and Words to Comfort

These practices are the same as those for other mainline Christians (see Chapter 21).

Bibliography

Association of Religion Data Archives. (n.d.). *Religious groups: Reformed/ Presbyterian*. Retrieved from http://www.thearda.com/denoms/ families/F_91.asp

Fowler, M. D. M. (2012). Presbyterians and others in the reformed tradition. In E. J. Taylor (Ed.), *Religion: A clinical guide for nurses* (pp. 233–240). New York, NY: Springer Publishing.

World Council of Churches. (n.d.). *Reformed churches*. Retrieved from https://www.oikoumene.org/en/church-families/reformed-churches

17

Christianity: Quaker (Friends)

Other Names and Similar Religious Traditions

The **Society of Friends** are often known as **Quakers** because of purported shaking—quaking—that occurred when they fervently explained their beliefs to those persecuting them centuries ago. There are four expressions of Quakerism: Programmed, Evangelical, Unprogrammed, and Conservative. Quakerism is considered one of the European Free Churches, also called Historic Peace churches.

Social and Historical Background

The Religious Society of Friends originated in the 1650s in England. Its founder was influenced by Anabaptist theology (see Chapter 5). Although there is no formalized creed, a central tenet is that there is something of God (i.e., "that of God") in everyone. This presence of God in all persons is also referred to as the Inner Light—or Divine Presence or Seed or Inward Teacher. This tenet explains Friends' aversion to killing anyone and weak or absent reliance on clergy. While many Friends would consider themselves Christian, many do not.

Among the Friends, there are several subgroups: Evangelical and "pastored" or "programmed" Friends have clergy, worship, and theology much like other Protestants; their services may include a short period of silence. Conservative and liberal "unprogrammed" Friends have a lay leader and worship in silence, awaiting the Holy Spirit's promptings to speak or sing. Liberals are extremely inclusive of diverse beliefs, as are conservatives to a lesser degree.

Worship and Devotional Practices

On Sundays, unprogrammed Friends will convene in a "meeting," while programmed Friends attend church. Regular business meetings are also scheduled. Whereas evangelical Friends view the Bible as inerrant and authoritative, liberal Friends accept there are multiple sources of sacred wisdom. Most Friends, however, are in the middle of this continuum. For those who do read the Bible, there is an emphasis on having the Holy Spirit guide the reading. Quakers understand the sacraments of baptism and communion to be internal, spiritual commitments and generally do not practice them outwardly.

A meditational approach to prayer is rather distinctive to Quakers. Meditation may begin with "retirement," a centering and being present in the moment. Prayer involves being more fully aware of God or the bigger reality; this can happen in meditation, in expressive artistry, or in living daily life. Evangelical Friends encourage families to pray and praise God every day. Thus:

- Given the diversity of prayer experiences among Quakers, when a patient indicates prayer with a nurse would be welcome, assess how the patient prefers to pray. Support or join, as appropriate. Prayer could involve sitting in worshipful silence together.
- Free Quaker devotional resources, such as readings, podcasts, and short videos, are available online at the *Friends Journal* (www.friendsjournal.org) and *QuakerSpeak* (quakerspeak.com).

Illness and Healing: Beliefs and Practices

There are no unique health-related beliefs or practices. Evangelicals believe in praying for healing but recognize that God may answer with spiritual rather than physical healing.

Beginning of Life: Beliefs and Practices

For evangelical Friends, all life is sacred, and induced abortion is opposed. Other Friends may not agree.

End of Life: Beliefs and Practices

Friends are diverse in their beliefs about afterlife. Evangelical Friends believe that at death the body "returns to dust" and that there is a judgment after Christ returns, and those who are righteous will live in God's presence forever, whereas the unrighteous will be separated from God and tormented by their evil. Some Friends, however, do not believe in any heaven or hell. Friends may even take pride in not focusing on the unknowable future, and rather focus on the present.

A Quaker funeral likely will be a simple service following a Sunday meeting. Cremation is preferred. Thus:

- Attempts to comfort by suggesting the dead are now with Christ would likely be inappropriate in some cases. Describing the deceased as "at Peace" or resting on the "other side" would always be appropriate.

Diet and Lifestyle: Prescriptions and Proscriptions

Tobacco, alcohol, illicit drugs, and other unwholesome habits are avoided.

Additional Miscellaneous Nursing Implications

- Friends' religious beliefs and practices are varied. Assess.

Ways and Words to Comfort

- For Friends, "go into the Light" and remembering that "all will be well" are characteristic comforting admonitions. Advice that grounds a Friend includes "let your life speak" (meaning, act on your beliefs).
- When making a decision, it is helpful to consider whether one is using his or her gifts to follow the light within and which choice will allow him or her to serve others.

Bibliography

Evangelical Friends Church Eastern Region. (2013). *Faith and practice: The book of discipline*. Retrieved from http://efcer.org/media/1/9/Faith-and-Practice-2013.pdf

Fager, C. E. (1996). *The authenticity of Liberal Quakerism*. Retrieved from https://universalistfriends.org/library/the-authenticity-of-liberal-quakerism?ref=library-list

Friends World Committee for Consultation. (n.d.). *Kinds of Friends*. Retrieved from http://fwcc.world/kinds-of-friends

18

Christianity: Restorationist

Other Names and Similar Religious Traditions

The Stone-Campbell **Restorationist** family of Christian churches include (1) the **Christian Churches and Churches of Christ**, (2) the **Christian Church (Disciples of Christ)**, and (3) the informal association of **Churches of Christ** (acapella or noninstrumental).

Social and Historical Background

These three branches have roots in 18th-century United Kingdom and early 19th-century United States. In response to the many subdivisions of Christianity, the American church founders were convinced that Christians should be more ecumenical and unified; they believed that this unity could be achieved by restoring the pattern of faith and organization of the early Christian church as described in the New Testament, and noninstrumental churches of Christ may even use lowercase "c" as a rejection of denominationalism. Congregations within Christian Church and Churches of Christ (noninstrumental) are loosely affiliated; each congregation self-governs.

Worship and Devotional Practices

A simple worship style is observed in weekly Sunday services that include communion. Churches of Christ (noninstrumental) use only unaccompanied singing during worship. Bible reading is emphasized. More contemporary worship styles (e.g., with worship team leading praise songs), however, are experienced in Christian Churches and Churches of Christ. For those unable to attend:

- Podcasts and videos of numerous local church services are available under Resources at Christian Church Today's website (cctoday.com).
- Local churches are available to bring Sunday communion to members.

Because these religious traditions are akin to other Christian denominations, see Chapter 21 for nursing implications.

Illness and Healing: Beliefs and Practices

Beliefs and practices regarding illness and healing are much like those of other mainstream Christians (see Chapter 21).

Beginning of Life: Beliefs and Practices

Given belief that baptism is by immersion and for those who understand its meaning as a symbol of incorporation into the life of Christ, there is no infant baptism (see also Chapter 21).

End of Life: Beliefs and Practices

Members of the Churches of Christ believe that if they leave the church, they can lose their salvation (see also Chapter 21).

Diet and Lifestyle: Prescriptions and Proscriptions

These practices are similar to those of other mainstream Christians (see Chapter 21).

Additional Miscellaneous Nursing Implications

- The Disciples of Christ sponsor the National Benevolent Association (NBA, n.d.), which organizes ministries for combating mental health stigma and for advocating and providing spiritual care for those in prison (and their families). The NBA also provides "back office" support for the over 40 locally based health and social justice ministries (e.g., support for homeless, abused, and indigent). Consult www.nbacares .org/partners-directory to determine what ministries may be in your area.
- Church members are often close-knit communities, willing to provide physical support to each other.

Ways and Words to Comfort

See Chapter 21.

Bibliography

Christ Church/Disciples of Christ. (n.d.). *History of the disciples.* Retrieved from https://disciples.org/our-identity/history-of-the-disciples

Gordon, B. (2016). *Churches of Christ.* Retrieved from https://www.namb.net/apologetics-blog/churches-of-christ

Lawson, L. (n.d.). *Who we are.* Retrieved from http://cctoday.com/who

National Benevolent Association. (n.d.). *NBA connect ministries.* Retrieved from https://www.nbacares.org/connect-ministries

Williams, D. N., Foster, D. A., & Blowers, P. M. (Eds.). (2013). *The Stone-Campbell Movement: A global history.* Danvers, MA: Chalice Press.

World Council of Churches. (n.d.). *Disciples of Christ/Churches of Christ.* Retrieved from https://www.oikoumene.org/en/church-families/disciples-of-christ-churches-of-christ

19

Christianity: Roman and Eastern Catholic

Other Names and Similar Religious Traditions

Roman Catholic is usually abbreviated as Catholic. Catholics include **Roman Catholics** (98%) and **Eastern Catholics** (2%)—formerly "rites," which are a communion of 23 distinct churches that developed within geographic locations and cultures.

Social and Historical Background

Roman Catholicism (originating in Western Europe), Eastern Catholicism, and Christian Orthodox churches (initially growing in Eastern Europe, the Middle East, Egypt, India, China, and Italy) are the oldest Christian traditions. During the Great Schism of 1054, the Eastern Christian church split with Rome and became known as Eastern Orthodox. At varying times in history, segments of these churches reunited with the Roman Catholic church to comprise the Eastern Catholic traditions.

Christianity developed in the first century, with the immediate followers of Jesus Christ as its original leaders, or apostles. Catholics believe that Jesus—the Son of God and a historical person—was miraculously birthed to the Virgin Mary and lived a life whereby he transformed people through teaching and healing (including regiving life to recently deceased). In his early 30s, he was crucified, buried, and resurrected. Jesus's life, death, and resurrection are redemptive, making it possible for all persons to be saved from sin and to be able to live eternally with God. Like most other Christians, Catholics believe in a Trinitarian God (i.e., God as Father, Son, and Holy Spirit).

Roman and Eastern Catholics accept the Pope as leader of the church; the Pope, along with the Magisterium (council of bishops), has the authority to define the doctrines of the church. Roman and Eastern Catholics share the same faith and have the same seven sacraments but have different customs and traditions that date back to the early centuries of the church. Roman and Eastern Catholics also place considerable weight on the authority of the church to guide believers' lives and influence their salvation. Today, the Roman Catholic church is the largest Christian faith tradition. Roughly one out of five Americans is Roman Catholic.

Worship and Devotional Practices

Worshipping God in community at church is a salient aspect of Catholic life. They worship following a liturgy (prayers and readings) that was translated from ancient Latin into the language of the worshipper. Catholics observe seven sacraments (signs that build faith and holiness), including communion. Indeed, communion is to be preceded by Penance (or Reconciliation or Confession), to receive the forgiveness of sins for serious sin or anytime the conscience is burdened. Receiving communion is central to church services (i.e., Mass [Roman], Divine Liturgy [Eastern]), and partaking of the bread and wine is believed to allow one to literally incorporate the body and blood of Christ. Beginning around the age of 7, members receive the Sacrament of Penance (Confession) and Holy Communion or Eucharist (for Roman Catholics; for Eastern Catholics, this begins in infancy); others can approach the priest during communion to receive a blessing. Members are obliged to receive Confession and Holy Communion at least once a year (preferably during Easter). They are encouraged to receive Communion every Sunday and on feast days—or daily, as long as they are in a state without mortal sin. Otherwise, Confession is a prerequisite. Thus:

- See Chapter 21 for communion-related health information.
- Devout patients unable to attend Mass will be eager to receive communion from a Eucharistic minister who can bring it to them. Per patient wishes, contact the chaplain or local parish.
- Communion wine is not offered outside of Mass. Holy Eucharist is considered complete when the bread ("host," usually a thin wheat wafer that can dissolve in the mouth) is consumed. If someone cannot consume wheat, partaking in only the sacramental wine is acceptable. Catholic chaplains, deacons, religious sisters, and lay Eucharistic Ministers typically distribute Holy Communion to hospital patients who wish to receive and are not nil per os (nothing by mouth, or NPO).

- Communion is to be preceded by at least a 1-hour fast (except for water); the sick and elderly, however, are exempt.
- Sunday is a weekly holy day for rest; members are encouraged to pursue family, cultural, and religious endeavors. Consult with patients as to how they prefer to observe "the Lord's Day."
- Sunday Masses are televised in most regions. Eternal Word Television Network (EWTN), available via cable or Internet, is a global Catholic network that offers daily Mass and prayers.

Other holy days celebrate important events in the life of Jesus or Mary. Particularly important is the 40-day season of Lent, from Ash Wednesday to Easter, when one self-examines and seeks purity of heart in preparation to celebrate Jesus's resurrection (Easter). Thus:

- Ash Wednesday and Good Friday are days of fasting and abstinence. That is, 18- to 59-year-olds abstain from meat and do not have solid foods between light meals (fasting). Abstinence from meat is to be observed every Friday of Lent; fish and dairy products are typically the proteins eaten instead. Illness at any age, however, is a reason for a dispensation from fasting.
- It is customary to identify something to do during Lent to build spiritual strength (e.g., to give up desserts or engage in Bible study or works of mercy).
- For Eastern Catholics, Lent begins two days earlier, on "Pure Monday" preceding Ash Wednesday. They observe a "strict fast" from meat and dairy products on the first day of Lent and on Good Friday. Abstinence from meat is practiced on Wednesdays and Fridays. Some Eastern Catholics observe stricter fasting practices like Orthodox Christians, also restricting such foods as fish, oil, and wine.

The sacrament of Anointing of the Sick is to receive the forgiveness of sins to bring spiritual healing and comfort and, if it is God's will, physical healing as well. Catholics believe that while only God can forgive human sins, Jesus also gave the apostles (and now passed down to priests through apostolic succession) the power to forgive sins. Thus:

- Appreciate the need to secure a priest to receive a patient's confession, if requested. This is especially important for the dying, who may request last rites (or extreme unction or viaticum). The family may be too overwhelmed to remember to call the priest, so the nurse can inquire and call a priest if chaplain services are unavailable.

Catholics also experience God when praying, meditating, almsgiving (doing charitable deeds), and reading inspirational material, including the Catholic Bible (which has some books not found in a Protestant Bible). They venerate Mary and the saints; that is, these individuals are asked to intercede with God/Jesus on behalf of the believer. The rosary (prayer beads that provide prompts for repetition of certain ritual prayers) is a common aid to prayer. A novena is a petitionary prayer repeated nine times in some pattern (e.g., nine Sundays in a row). Thus:

- When a Catholic requests prayer, any Christian style will be appreciated. A memorized or read prayer or silent meditational prayer will likely be comfortable.
- Treat any rosaries, icons, or other religious objects with respect; keep them where the patient wants them.

Illness and Healing: Beliefs and Practices

Given the age of this tradition, it is not surprising that Catholics have studied bioethical issues extensively. Several principles guide a Catholic approach to healthcare decisions: (1) defer moral decisions to church teachings; (2) respect the dignity of all persons; (3) be good stewards, or responsible guardians, of life; (4) remember life is sacred from conception; and (5) support social justice. Thus:

- Organ transplantation is considered a gift one gives to humanity.
- Gene therapy (or any therapy) is permitted if the integrity and dignity of the person is not harmed. Genetic material, however, ought not be derived from embryonic stem cells.

Like other Christians, Catholics can interpret health challenges in many ways. They may, however, be more apt to ascribe meaning to suffering by remembering the modeling of Jesus on the cross.

The Sacrament of the Sick, historically performed just at the end of life (and called Last Rites), is now available for any who are physically, mentally, or spiritually sick or disabled. It is often offered prior to surgery. Thus:

- Be cautious when inquiring of an older Catholic patient if he or she would like prayer or anointing, as it could be misinterpreted as indicating the clinician thinks he or she will die soon.
- If the Catholic is gravely ill, it would be appropriate to offer to contact a priest (or request the chaplain do so) so that the Sacrament of the Sick may be received.

Beginning of Life: Beliefs and Practices

The purposes of sexual intercourse are union and procreation. Because these purposes are inseparable and only God has dominion over human bodies, a number of beliefs and practices result: (1) artificial contraception is not to be practiced; (2) masturbation, because it is experienced outside the union between a man and woman, is unacceptable; and (3) sterilization, surrogacy, in vitro fertilization, sex selection, donor insemination, and artificial insemination (unless it assists with fertilization) are morally impermissible. Because life begins at conception, abortion would be killing. Prenatal testing is only appropriate if the intent is to safeguard the patients or promote health. If the child had a life-limiting condition, the parents may choose to forgo aggressive treatment, opting instead for nutrition and palliative care. Thus:

- Given many Catholics disagree with some of these teachings, it is important to assess parental preferences. Likewise, given the teachings, Catholics who go against them may experience guilt, shame, or family conflict. For such, spiritual care expertise (e.g., chaplain) will be beneficial.
- Baptism is normally administered shortly after birth or when in danger of death. If there is any possibility that an infant or young child may die without yet having been baptized (e.g., stillborn), ask the parents if they desire the Sacrament of Baptism for their child. Although a priest is preferred, in an emergency, anyone with the right intention may do so. If a nurse is needed and so inclined, an appropriate baptism would involve pouring tap water (or holy or blessed water, if available) over the child's head three times while saying, "I baptize you in the name of the Father [pour], the Son [pour], and Holy Spirit [pour]. Amen."

End of Life: Beliefs and Practices

Death marks the end of a person's earthly pilgrimage and is the gateway to eternal life with God. The soul is believed to separate from the body at death; it is immediately judged. Those whose faith and works indicate acceptance of God's grace will go to heaven—"the fulfillment of the deepest human longings"—the place where one lives with the Trinity, Mary, angels, and others who are so blessed (U.S. Catholic Church, 2003, p. 1024). Going to heaven will either be immediate (for those whose souls are pure enough to live in the presence of God) or after a process of purification (purgatory). The unconverted, or those who die without repenting a grave sin, will go to an eternal separation from God (hell). At an unknown time, Christ will return, the dead will be raised to life (and the body and soul will be reunited), and a Last Judgment will reveal the good or evil of each person. After this, the righteous will live with God in a renewed universe. Thus:

- Believers are encouraged to prepare for their death; receiving a final forgiveness and commendation from a priest just prior to death is vital. Nurses can make accommodation for this.
- Cremation is permitted as well as full body burial. Ashes may not be scattered on land or at sea.
- Autopsies are permitted.
- Donation of a body for medical research is permitted.
- Although suicide, assisted suicide, and active euthanasia are considered immoral, God does provide opportunity for repentance (U.S. Catholic Church, 2003, p. 2283).
- Any treatment for pain at the end of life (e.g., conscious sedation) is appropriate as long as it does not prevent the spiritual preparation for death.
- When the quality of a good life is outweighed by the burden of prolonging life, life-sustaining treatments can be withheld or withdrawn. A person is not obligated to use extraordinary means in preserving life, but basic nutrition and hydration should be provided if the benefit outweighs the burden to the involved.
- Advanced Directives are endorsed by the Catholic Church.
- Organ and tissue donations are permitted.
- There is no objection to blood transfusions or the use of blood products.

Diet and Lifestyle: Prescriptions and Proscriptions

Catholics have no dietary restrictions. See "Worship and Devotional Practices" regarding fasting practices (e.g., 1-hour fast prior to receiving Communion).

Additional Miscellaneous Nursing Implications

- In North America, there is a shortage of priests. Thus, those visiting a patient may be ordained deacons, sisters, or laypeople. While these persons can bring communion, only a priest can offer the Sacrament of the Sick.
- Some Catholics may wear a scapular around their neck; this necklace-like amulet is a symbol of devotion, but sometimes it is misconstrued to be a guarantee of salvation. Surgical patients wearing a scapular will not want to remove it; it can be taped to their body away from the operative site.
- The National Catholic Bioethics Center is available for consultation. Requests can be emailed via their website: www.ncbcenter.org.

Ways and Words to Comfort

- Reading of sacred scripture or other devotional material especially the following Bible passages: Psalm 121, Psalm 91:1–9, Psalm 23, 2 Corinthians 1:3–6.
- Listening to religious music or watching televised worship services.
- Arrange for Catholic Holy Communion, Confession, or Sacrament of the Sick, if desired.
- Welcome to the bedside symbols of faith such as icons, rosaries, or crucifixes.
- Churches invite members to submit their names for prayer by those attending services; sometimes this is done by writing a prayer request in a prayer book. Catholics can find comfort in remembering that fellow members are praying for them.
- Healing and comforting prayers include:
  - The Blessing of Aaron (see the appendix).
  - Prayer of God's Presence ("*God, my Father, You have promised to remain forever with those who do what is just and right. Help me to live in Your presence. The loving plan of Your Wisdom was made known when Jesus, Your Son, became man like us. I want to obey His commandment of love and bring Your peace and joy to others. Keep before me the wisdom and love You have made known in Your Son. Help me to be like Him in work and deed.*")
  - Our Father (see "Lord's Prayer" in the appendix).
  - Hail Mary ("*Hail Mary, full of Grace, the Lord is with thee. Blessed are thou among women and blessed is the fruit of thy womb, Jesus. Holy Mary, Mother of God, pray for us sinners now and at the hour of our death.*")
  - The Memorare ("*Remember, O most gracious Virgin Mary, that never was it known that anyone who fled to thy protection, implored thy help, or sought thy intercession, was left unaided. Inspired with this confidence, I fly unto thee, O virgin of virgins, my mother. To thee I come; before thee I stand, sinful and sorrowful. O mother of the Sword Incarnate, despise not my petitions; but in thy clemency, hear and answer me. Amen.*")

Bibliography

Donovan, C. B. (n.d.). *Catholic rites and churches*. EWTN: Global Catholic Network. Retrieved from http://www.ewtn.com/expert/answers/rites .htm

Dysinger, L. (2012). Roman Catholics. In E. J. Taylor (Ed.), *Religion: A clinical guide for nurses* (pp. 241–250). New York, NY: Springer Publishing.

Eastern Catholic Churches. (n.d.). *Eastern Catholic Churches.* Retrieved from https://www.catholicsandcultures.org/eastern-catholic-churches

Hamel, R. P., & O'Rourke, K. (2002). *The Roman Catholic tradition: Religious beliefs and healthcare decisions.* Chicago, IL: The Park Ridge Center. Retrieved from https://www.advocatehealth.com/assets/documents/faith/roman_catholic3.pdf

Our Catholic Prayers. (n.d.). *Some special prayers.* Retrieved from https://www.ourcatholicprayers.com/special-prayers.html

United States Catholic Conference. (1994). *Catechism of the Catholic Church* (2nd ed.). New York, NY: Doubleday.

U.S. Catholic Church. (2003). *Catechism of the Catholic Church* (2nd ed.). New York, NY: Doubleday.

U.S. Conference of Catholic Bishops. (n.d.). *Home.* Retrieved from http://www.usccb.org

20

Christianity: Seventh-Day Adventist

Other Names and Similar Religious Traditions

Offshoots of Seventh-Day Adventists (SDAs) include **Seventh-Day Adventist Reform Movement** (traditionalists) and **Free Seventh-Day Adventists** (African Americans). A few very small, but theologically similar, groups exist in the Adventist religion family.

Social and Historical Background

Seventh-Day Adventism is a Protestant denomination emerging from the mid-19th-century revival period in the United States. This is the group that interpreted the biblical books of Daniel and Revelation to mean that Christ would return in 1844 (and who survived this "Great Disappointment") and continued to search the Bible for understanding of when the return (advent) of Christ would be. This emphasis on an imminent "Second Coming" as well as a literal Sabbath keeping (learned from Seventh-Day Baptists) prompted the name for the denomination. One of the church's pioneers was Ellen G. White, a prolific author and viewed by most SDAs as a prophetess. Given the view that Christ's return is soon, SDAs actively evangelize their "end time message."

Worship and Devotional Practices

The Sabbath, kept from sundown Friday to sundown Saturday, is a distinctive time for these Christians. In addition to attending services at church, SDAs spend this sacred time resting from unnecessary work—enjoying family, fellowshipping with fellow members, and participating service-oriented or recreational activities. (The nature of what is thought to be appropriate Sabbath activity varies widely.) SDAs worship much like other nonliturgical Protestant Christians (see Chapter 21). Corporate worship on Saturday mornings is preceded by Sabbath School, a time for Bible study (available online at ssnet.org for all ages). SDAs often worship privately at the start of the day and/or end of the day (i.e., pray and read the Bible, Sabbath School lesson, Ellen White writings, or other inspirational material). Traditional families may also do this as a family. Thus:

- Ascertain how the patient would like to "keep Sabbath." Unnecessary treatments and procedures will likely be avoided. Assist the patient to have a restful and spiritually invigorating environment (e.g., provide Christian music, turn television off).
- Protect and support, if needed, the patient's devotional time (e.g., prevent interruptions, provide quietness, bring requested reading material).
- SDA-run media include the Hope Channel, Three Angels Broadcasting Network (3ABN), Loma Linda Broadcasting Network (LLBN), and Adventist World Radio. These, as well as other Christian media, will likely be beneficial to the homebound SDA.

Illness and Healing: Beliefs and Practices

The rationales for living healthfully and theological interpretations for health mirror those of other Protestant faiths. Likewise, critically ill SDAs may request anointing (see Chapter 21).

The SDA "Health Message" was influenced by the American health reformers of the late 19th century and is described in Ellen White's writings (see "Diet and Lifestyle"). This Health Message is the impetus not only for health promotion activities within the church but also for the health promotion and healthcare endeavors the church conducts around the world.

Beginning of Life: Beliefs and Practices

There are no distinctions from other Protestant Christians (see Chapter 21).

End of Life: Beliefs and Practices

Death and burial practices are similar to those of other Protestant Christians. Death is metaphorically described as being asleep and the body returning "dust to dust." SDAs do not believe they go immediately to heaven; rather, at the Second Coming of Jesus, all are resurrected. A final judgment is held, and those who have committed themselves to God will be granted eternal life (in heaven and then later in an "earth made new"). Those who do not want to be with God will permanently die in a hell that is not eternal. Thus:

- Comforting words for those experiencing death emphasize the hope of a Second Coming (e.g., "The next thing he will see is Jesus's coming" or "She is peacefully asleep now" or "We are waiting for the Lord's return"), instead of the classic Christian comfort of the deceased "being with Jesus now."

Diet and Lifestyle: Prescriptions and Proscriptions

SDAs have long touted a lacto-ovo vegetarian diet (although the more conservative may now be vegans). They also promote a holistic approach to health, advocating not only vegetarianism, exercise, sunshine and fresh air, adequate sleep, hydration, and abstinence from harmful substances (tobacco, alcohol, illicit drugs), but also trust in divine power (God). Although many SDAs are not vegetarian, these SDAs will still refrain from the "unclean" meats listed in the Old Testament (e.g., pork, shellfish). Thus:

- Assess for what diet and other health-promoting strategies (listed in the previous paragraph) the patient desires.

Additional Miscellaneous Nursing Implications

- SDA churches often have a "Health and Temperance Committee"; such a committee is charged with promoting health within the congregation and/or wider community. Public health ventures can tap this resource.
- Deaconesses (elected, untrained women in the church) may provide informal caregiving support to members.
- In large congregations, an Adventist Community Services Center ("Dorcas Society") may exist to provide services such as giving used clothing and domestic items to anyone in the neighborhood.

Ways and Words to Comfort

- Respect the patient's desires regarding keeping Sabbath; when greeting the SDA patient near the start of the Sabbath, it would be appropriate to wish them a "Happy Sabbath!"
- At appropriate times, an offer of a colloquial prayer would likely be welcomed (see Chapter 21). SDAs like to think of prayer "as talking to a Friend."

Bibliography

Byrd, A. (2015). *Seventh-day Adventist Reform Movement president explains century old church split*. Retrieved from https://spectrummagazine.org/article/2015/04/11/seventh-day-adventist-reform-movement-president-explains-century-old-church-split

Carr, M. (2012). Seventh-day Adventists. In E. J. Taylor (Ed.), *Religion: A clinical guide for nurses* (pp. 251–256). New York, NY: Springer Publishing.

DuBose, E. R., & Walters, J. W. (2002). *The Seventh-day Adventist tradition: Religious beliefs and healthcare decisions.* Chicago, IL: The Park Ridge Center. Retrieved from https://www.advocatehealth.com/assets/documents/faith/adventist3.pdf

General Conference of Seventh-day Adventists. (n.d.-a). *Beliefs*. Retrieved from https://www.adventist.org/en/beliefs

General Conference of Seventh-day Adventists. (n.d.-b). *History*. Retrieved from https://www.adventist.org/en/information/history

International Association of Free Seventh-day Adventists. (2018). *The Free SDA movement today.* Retrieved from http://www.freesda.org/history/freesdastoday.html

Sahlin, M. (2018). *Adventist denominations: The larger picture.* Adventist Today. Retrieved from https://atoday.org/adventist-denominations-the-larger-picture

Seventh-day Adventist Reform Movement president explains century old church split. (2015). Retrieved from https://spectrummagazine.org/article/2015/04/11/seventh-day-adventist-reform-movement-president-explains-century-old-church-split

21

Christianity: Unspecified

Other Names and Similar Religious Traditions

Christian, **Protestant**, **interdenominational**, and **nondenominational** are all terms some patients will use to self-describe. These Christians can be **evangelical** (typified by missionary or social reform, "born again" conversion, emphasis on the "good news" of Jesus's salvation, and a view of the Bible as the ultimate authority); **fundamentalist** (characterized by theological conservativism and acceptance of the Bible as historically accurate); or **charismatic** (known for an emphasis on the work of the Holy Spirit). Some interor nondenominational congregations are a "**community church.**"

Social and Historical Background

Many Christians who are firmly attached to a denomination may prefer to self-describe as Christian before their denominational affiliation. This could be to signify their membership of the worldwide Church. Others who so self-identify, however, may not be engaged within a particular denomination, although they may have been earlier in life. They may be a "hyphenated" Christian who finds benefit from multiple denominations, or they may resist denominational affiliation for a theological or personal reason. For example, they may be frustrated with traditional Christian institutions, yet they may be actively engaged in a house or café church. Or they may belong to a traditional congregation that purposefully is noncreedal and loosely affiliated with other such churches. Although a Roman Catholic could self-identify as simply "Christian," it is more likely that someone from a Protestant background will.

There are a variety of reasons for being nondenominational; however, the commonality is the adherence to the most essential of Christian beliefs. For example, these believers likely will accept a Trinitarian God. God, the Father, created all and is the source of love. God's Son, Jesus (the Christ), born in ancient Israel (c. 6–4 BCE), was the personification of God. His life, death on a cross, and resurrection (c. 31–33 CE) demonstrated divine love and purposed to provide humanity an expiation or atonement for sins (i.e., reconciliation of humanity to God). God's Holy Spirit, an invisible comforter and guide, when invited, is present to empower the believer to live out God's will.

Christians generally accept the Old and New Testaments of the Bible (and possibly some extra ancient books) as sacred scripture. There are variations of belief, however, about its inerrancy and methods for interpretation. Indeed, these variations are what typically explain the thousands (or hundreds—depending on the source) of Christian denominations.

Worship and Devotional Practices

Some Christians follow the liturgical calendar (which identifies what Bible passages to read each day and when to celebrate holy events). Well-known holidays include Christmas (to celebrate Jesus's birth) and Easter (Jesus's resurrection from the dead) when believers typically attend church and celebrate with a family meal. Lent (the 40 days prior to Easter) may be a time of heightened spiritual discipline (e.g., fasting). Thus:

- Committed Christians likely have a devotional time each day (often early mornings), when they read the Bible or religious material and pray. For hospitalized patients, nurses can protect this time from intrusions.
- Some patients wishing to fast from food may need consultation (e.g., those with diabetes, eating disorders). Given that fasting is done not to earn God's love but to focus on it more, patients can be reminded to consider alternative means for achieving that purpose (e.g., fasting from other things that distract one from God or fasting from processed and unhealthful foods or drink).

Community worship is usually on Sunday mornings, with additional options at large churches possibly being available Saturday or Sunday evenings. A Sunday evening and midweek church service (e.g., "prayer meeting") may also be frequented. Thus:

- If a church member cannot continue to attend services, this likely creates a social and spiritual void. Most denominations have large congregations that live-stream their services, if not television programming, that can partially fill the void. These are often archived on the church's website.

- Many churches have clergy or laypersons who visit the sick and may provide some support. These resources cannot be mobilized, however, if the church does not know about the patient's condition. Because some patients may not want fellow congregants to know of their illness or disability, the wise nurse will always ask the patient before mobilizing church resources.
- Many congregations have "prayer chains" through which they encourage the congregation to pray for the sick, as well as healing services where prayers are offered for those requesting them.
- Many denominations employ cell or growth groups forming tighter, more intimate communities within the larger church fellowship. This affords a family atmosphere of caring and support capturing many congregants before they "fall through the cracks" when ill or in crisis.

Protestant Christian churches generally practice the sacraments (the outer expression of an inner grace from God) of baptism and communion. Whereas some Christians baptize infants and children, others wait until an age of understanding. Some baptize with sprinkling water on the head; others will immerse the head or body. The frequency of celebration of Communion (or the Lord's Supper or Eucharist) varies. It involves the partaking of bread (or a wafer or cracker) and wine (or grape juice), which may be preceded by feet washing, to commemorate Jesus's final meal before his crucifixion. The frequency of this important ritual varies, with some practicing it every week, while most do it monthly, quarterly, or annually. Thus:

- If communion is desired by the hospitalized or homebound patient, contact the healthcare organization's chaplain, who can then contact the church—if the family has not yet done so.
- For patients who are nil per os (nothing by mouth, or NPO), a blessing can be spoken by the officiant in lieu of ingesting the communion elements.
- For those who cannot consume the wine or wheat-based bread for health reasons, it is acceptable not to take that which is deleterious. Alternatively, one can request grape juice instead of wine or a gluten-free wafer. (Give ample notice, however.)
- Likewise, those with compromised immune systems who ought to avoid drinking from a chalice (communal cup) can request it be served in an individual cup (prior to any service).

Prayer is an intentional way of deepening one's relationship with God. Christian prayer typically involves verbally or silently talking to God and reflection and quietness to listen to God's response. For some, a ritual or read prayer is more comfortable. Bible study or meditating on a passage of Scripture, especially the Psalms, can also be prayer. More unconventional Protestant approaches to prayer include journal writing, expressive art (e.g., drawing, poetry, singing, dancing), and use of imagery. The quintessential prayer of the Christian is the "Lord's Prayer" (recorded in the biblical book of Matthew); its phrase "thy will be done on earth as it is in heaven" indicates to Christians that prayer is about co-orienting oneself with God. Thus:

- When patients become ill, they may pray more fervently, or they may find praying becomes difficult (e.g., because they cannot concentrate or because they are angry at God). Discussing difficulties and learning novel ways to pray while sick can be helpful; therefore, facilitate a connection with a spiritual director or other spiritual care expert if the patient so desires.
- If objective data indicate it is appropriate, inquire if they would like you or other clinicians of faith to pray (e.g., ask, "Would a prayer be helpful?").
- Alternatively, use an indicator (e.g., wear a lapel pin with praying hands, a framed quote about prayer hung in a clinic room or office) to show your receptivity toward prayer. (Note: Confirm this is legal and approved where you work. For example, in many European countries, this would not be allowed. In a government-funded U.S. American hospital, it could be construed as a threat to the First Amendment.)
- If a patient requests prayer, a willing nurse with even a smidgeon of shared belief can use the formula for colloquial prayer used by many Christian nurses:
  - Open (identify divine listener)—for example, "Dear God" or "Our Father" or "Lord."
  - *Set the stage (connect with the here and now)—for example, "Susie is about to go to surgery, and we are anxious . . ." or "Life is difficult right now for Lee, with worries about his family, his health, his finances. . . ."
  - Request (link perceived needs with how God can help)—for example, "Please assist the surgical team, and grace Susie with inner peace as she goes to the operating room. . . ."
  - *Wrap up (prepare for closing)—for example, "We know you hear and answer us; we are so thankful for your grace and mercy."
  - Close (signal the end of prayer)—for example, "Your will be done; amen" or "In Christ's name, amen."
  [* Not all nurses include these second and fourth elements.]
  If possible, however, a nurse should first assess how the patient prefers to pray and try to accommodate (e.g., "How do you usually pray?" "In what way would you like me to pray now?")

- If a patient requests prayer, also ask the patient for what they would like prayer for (e.g., "What you like me to pray about?"). This will provide insight about what concerns are most important. It can also function as a springboard for deeper discourse that may be therapeutic.

- Intercessory prayer, a type of prayer, involves petitioning God for a specific request (e.g., for a cure, safety, restored relationship). When such a prayer is appropriate, pray to invite God's will and understand it will manifest in the way that is ultimately best (e.g., "God, we want a cure for this cancer and relief from this pain; yet we ask You to open our hearts to Your loving will to be done").

- If uncomfortable with an extemporaneous prayer, a read prayer (see the appendix) will also comfort the Christian patient. Although some Christians may feel uncomfortable with it, a few moments of shared silence offered with respect and compassion can be helpful (e.g., "I'd love to pray with you yet don't feel comfortable speaking it; would you be okay with me sitting with you in silent prayer for a few moments?").

- When in pain or extremis, it is difficult to pray in a colloquial manner. Instead, a repetitive short phrase will likely be helpful (e.g., "Lord, have mercy!" or "Live out Your love within me" or "Jesus loves me" or "Come, Lord Jesus!").

- If a patient feels that he or she is not "good enough" or not praying "well enough" to be healed, this may indicate a spiritual crisis that needs expert attention. Given congregational ministers typically have minimal training in counseling, referral to a trained chaplain is likely best. A wise nurse will follow up on the referral and inquire how the patient feels after the intervention.

- **Never coerce prayer.** Obtain permission; inquire in a way that allows the patient to comfortably refuse. If the patient refuses, do not repeat the offer later. After a refusal, however, you can "leave the door open" (e.g., "No worries. If you ever would like me to pray with you, know that I'll be happy to"). Remember, you can always pray privately for a patient. Furthermore, the rapport and relationship you build with a patient can be the best prompt for a patient request for prayer.

Illness and Healing: Beliefs and Practices

Most Christians believe they were created by God (albeit they disagree about the process of creation). Therefore, God can recreate and heal. Christians typically view their bodies as "temples of God"; that is, they are vessels for God's Spirit to live and work. Accordingly, one is to steward it respectfully (e.g., pursue a healthful lifestyle, seek healthcare when it is needed). Thus:

- These beliefs have implications for motivating patients to make healthful choices. Motivational interviewing, without imposing guilt, can be enriched by tapping this worldview.

Disease and disability are often interpreted as the results of sin, whether it be a personal sin (e.g., personal actions, stress) or being part of a sinful world (e.g., pathogens, pollution, inaccessible health-care). Although the Christian's response can be to doubt and distance oneself from God, suffering can also prompt spiritual transformation. Indeed, a Christian view of suffering includes how it is a crucible that allows persons to draw closer to God. Thus:

- Nurses are in a pivotal position to nudge persons with illness and disability to positively reframe their struggles. For Christians, reframing can include interpreting a health challenge as an opportunity to grow closer to God.
- For patients experiencing anger at God, acknowledge that this is common and normal, and encourage a referral to an expert (e.g., spiritual director, chaplain, psychologist).

Healing comes from the Great Physician (God) but is often mediated by healthcare providers. Christians pray, find consolation in fellow believers, and, when quite sick, often request anointing, unction, or a "ministration of the sick." Regardless of denomination, this ritual involves religious leader(s) laying hands on the patient, anointing with oil (usually the forehead or hands), and praying; the patient may be encouraged to reflect and seek repentance prior to the service. Thus:

- When such a ritual occurs at the hospital bedside, nurses can prepare not only the patient and room to receive extra visitors but also the guests who may be disturbed by the severity of the patient's physical condition. Encourage visitors to talk, pray, or read the Bible to the patient in a normal voice even if the patient cannot talk.
- It is also not unusual for patients who perceive a nurse as safe, to "confess" their sins to them (e.g., by telling painful stories of their past or making statements like, "God will never forgive me"). An appropriate nurse response is to use empathic listening (e.g., let the patient talk, create responses that attempt to name their feelings, and prompt them to reflect). Per patient request, a referral can be made for spiritual care experts or clergy who can offer a ritual to symbolize forgiveness.

Beginning of Life: Beliefs and Practices

Generally, Protestant Christians believe in abstinence until marriage, and use of contraception is acceptable. Abortion, however, is typically not condoned, unless the mother's life is threatened. Circumcision is often practiced, but not for religious reasons (see also Chapter 19).

End of Life: Beliefs and Practices

Although there are variations in beliefs about what happens after death, Christians believe that because Jesus conquered death (as he was resurrected after a gruesome death and returned to heaven), there is an afterlife. While some Christians describe an immediate reunion of the soul with God after death, others believe the reunion of the righteous occurs after a return of Jesus when there will be a resurrection of the body and/or spirit, followed by a final judgment. The righteous will be with God; for most, this is in a "heaven" and then eternally in the world made new. The unrighteous, or those who would not want to be with God, will not be with God; this is variously interpreted to mean a literal and eternal hell, or an immediate destruction. Thus:

- Because life is a sacred gift from God, euthanasia and suicide are not condoned; however, Christians usually believe that nothing can separate them from the love (and forgiveness) of God.
- Organ donation is acceptable, if not encouraged.
- Increasingly, cremation is accepted.
- Although Christians have beliefs to assuage death-related anxiety, it is typical that they will still experience stress when considering their death. Supporting them to remember that anxiety—even for a Christian—is normal. Beliefs about heaven can provide comfort.
- For patients and family members, death-related anxiety and interpersonal tension may be generated by concern over whether one is "saved" or in the righteous camp. Such concerns may best be discussed with a spiritual care expert. The nurse, however, is the frontline listener who can assess and make a referral.
- Christian traditions typically do not have any special postmortem care practices. In some cultures, however, Christians may have specific rituals for bathing the deceased and burial.
- Several phrases may be used to describe what happens at death. The body may "return to dust"; the person may be "resting in the Lord" or having "soul sleep" or "have gone to be with the Lord." Given the diverse beliefs regarding what happens immediately after death, the nurse needs to be cautious in offering comforting

statements. For example, "Your loved one has gone to be with the Lord" may not be apropos for a family who does not believe this. Deeply listen as they explain what is comforting.

Diet and Lifestyle: Prescriptions and Proscriptions

- All Christian denominations would advocate for moderation, if not abstinence, from alcohol and tobacco. All would urge abstinence from illicit drugs; however, use of medical marijuana where it is illegal may prompt desire for discussion with clergy.
- Most devout Christians would pray a short prayer of gratitude prior to a meal. In some circumstances, it may be appropriate for a nurse to offer such a prayer (e.g., with young hospitalized children whose parents request it, for Christian patients with dementia who may find this reorienting).
- Extramarital intercourse and pornography would be sinful. Some denominations condone divorce, especially for those whose partner was unfaithful, while some do not.
- While many Christian doctrinal statements do not condone lesbian, gay, bisexual, transgender, and queer (LGBTQ) lifestyles and same-sex marriages, a few denominations do. All would agree, however, that LGBTQ persons are to be loved. How this love is expressed varies, with some Christians insisting the LGBTQ repress or convert their sexual orientation. Consequently, some LGBTQ patients will want nothing to do with their Christian past, while others may be deeply religious (e.g., see Chapter 13).

Additional Miscellaneous Nursing Implications

- Many Christian churches organize themselves to provide some social support to their ill members. These laypersons may make visits, bring food, provide spiritual solace, or meet other needs of the patient. Such groups include the Order of St. Luke (an ecumenical healing order composed of laity and clergy) and Stephen Ministry (a ministry training organization for laity; https://www.stephenministries.org/default.cfm); local church deacons and deaconesses may also provide support. Frequently, the Protestant churches have Sunday Schools, where members meet to study and pray together. Sunday School groups can be an important part of support to those who are ill by visiting, providing meals, arranging transportation, and performing other activities.
- Some larger congregations may have a paid or voluntary faith community nurse. Faith community nurses and congregational

health ministries are a valuable resource for providing spiritual support, health education, augmentation of discharge planning, and community resource and referral information. For further information, see the Westberg Institute for Faith Community Nursing's website at westberginstitute.org/faith -community-nursing.

- While members of some more conservative traditions may prefer only to have clergy from their denomination visit, some will be grateful for any clergy (i.e., minister, reverend, bishop, pastor) who visit. When clergy do visit, it may be helpful to prepare them for what to expect when they visit their parishioner; the nurse can also try to arrange care so that the visit is not interrupted.

Ways and Words to Comfort

- Most Christians use a colloquial style of prayer that is silent and solo. See the earlier section "Worship and Devotional Practices" for tips on how to offer prayer or respond to patient prayer requests.
- Bible reading is important. Particularly comforting Bible passages are listed in the appendix. If a nurse is asked to read from the Bible, familiar Scriptures that remind believers of God's love, acceptance, and presence during difficult times would be welcomed. It would be an affirmation of one's faith when fear and doubt might be felt.
- Religious music in a style preferred by the patient might be comforting (e.g., hymns, gospel music, spirituals, Christian contemporary, noninstrumental). YouTube renditions and websites with lyrics exist (e.g., opc.org/hymnal.html).

Bibliography

Pew Research Center. (2018). *Religious landscape study.* Retrieved from http://www.pewforum.org/religious-landscape-study

Taylor, E. J. (2003). Prayer's clinical issues and implications. *Holistic Nursing Practice, 17,* 179–188.

Taylor, E. J. (2012). *Religion: A clinical guide for nurses.* New York, NY: Springer Publishing.

22

Hinduism

Other Names and Similar Religious Traditions

Other names for Hinduism include **Sanatana Dharma** and **Vedic** religion. Four major Hindu divisions or varieties and numerous sects exist; many gurus have their own followings.

Social and Historical Background

The beginnings of Hinduism are traced to sacred texts written around 1700 BCE. It developed in the Indian subcontinent and reflects its many subcultures. There are no creeds, and there is much tolerance for a variety of beliefs. Although there is no organization governing the religion, several fundamentalist militant bodies have assumed control. Given these factors, there is much diversity of belief and practice, making the assessment of a Hindu patient's culture and religiosity all the more necessary.

Most Hindus believe in one ultimate reality or Absolute God (*Brahman*, or *Ishwar*); Brahman is manifested in thousands of gods or goddesses, just as a sun is reflected by rays. The gods or goddesses each reflect a certain characteristic of God (e.g., fertility, health, wisdom). Incarnated forms of God have lived on earth and are likewise worshipped. Another belief with implications for health is that of the cycle of rebirthing (reincarnation), where birth and death are time points when a soul enters or leaves a physical body. Principles that influence the life of a Hindu include purity of mind and body, self-control, detachment from worldly and personal things, truth, and nonviolence.

The purpose of life is to live such that the next life will achieve union with God, or ultimate liberation (moksha)—freedom from the human condition or a sense that all is one. While living as human, however, what happens is determined by actions and deeds of past lives (karma); likewise, what one does in the present life will determine what happens in the next life or lives. To reach moksha, Hindus follow the divine law or path of righteousness (dharma), which involves living virtuously and detaching from the world.

Other primary purposes for life include making a prosperous livelihood and pleasing the senses. Normally, individuals progress through four stages during a life span with rules and expectations in each. During youth, one develops and learns. During the generative years of adulthood, one marries, bears children, supports others, and so forth. During the retirement years, one gives back to the community and begins more actively to disengage from the world. In old age, one becomes more ascetic, preparing for moksha. While these four stages for the personal life provide ethical structure, the caste system provides social structure. The caste rules and obligations vary among the thousands of subcastes.

Worship and Devotional Practices

A Hindu can worship any representation of Brahman anywhere anytime. For some, the god Brahman is an intangible principle, whereas for others, Brahman is manifest in a pantheon of gods or goddesses that are ascribed human characteristics and can be petitioned, befriended, and cajoled with vows. A vow can be prescribed by a priest, learned in astrology, who functions like a shaman to calculate the best time and best ritual for the appropriate god or goddess. Thus, the timing, frequency, and rituals of worship may reflect what a priest has recommended. For example, a patient may perform a puja (religious ritual) a specified number of times during a time frame, pray a specified mantra selected by the priest, or fast or abstain from specified foods. Hinduism is not intrinsically a congregational religion; the temple exists for individuals as a place for performing religious rituals recommended by the priest. Doctrinal Hinduism (bhakti) is a spiritual movement led by gurus and other devout religious teachers outside the temple. Thus:

■ Although they are not expected to regularly visit a temple, Hindus in North America often do so on Sundays even though Tuesday is considered more auspicious by many Hindus. The day of the week that a person visits the temple may reflect what deity they are worshipping. Temple visits will likely also occur during a number of holy days or festivals or when a person wants to do a puja (e.g., to seek healing).

- Respect the Hindu patient's need for an astrological consult prior to a major procedure or travel (e.g., transfer home).

The purpose of religious rituals may be to worship or petition a deity or to develop spiritual discipline to achieve moksha. Rituals include recited, chanted, or sung mantras (prayers taken from sacred text); meditation (often involving the repeating of a mantra while sitting in the "lotus position"); and yoga (spiritual meditation for the purpose of self-realization and liberation that usually involves focusing on breathing while assuming a special posture). Worship may occur at home or a temple. A deity is often worshipped at a shrine that has a tangible image of that god or goddess; the worshipper may light a candle or offer the deity fruit or flowers. A devout Hindu may worship every morning at sunrise as well as noon and sunset. Most Hindus accept the oldest sacred writings, the Vedas; however, the Bhagavad Gita (or Gita) and Ramayana are other sacred texts that provide guidance for living. Vedic hymns are typically recited silently, softly, or in community at the beginning of new life adventures (e.g., birth, marriage). Thus:

- Be respectful of puja or rituals being implemented (e.g., a fast observed; not removing requisite jewelry or holy thread at the waist or wrist; not wiping off *tilaka* marks on the forehead or other parts of the body).
- Inquire if support for yogic practices are needed (e.g., schedule uninterrupted meditation time, assist with washing prior to prayer, make space for a shrine, play a YouTube recording of a healing mantra [e.g., Dhanvantari mantra for healing, at www .youtube.com/watch?v=w4m28Z5OyFk]).

Illness and Healing: Beliefs and Practices

How much patients hold traditional Indian Hindu beliefs about illness and healing will likely be associated with how culturally assimilated they are in a culture influenced by Western scientific beliefs. Traditionally, however, Hindus believe health is maintained when there is a balance of mind, body, and soul (which includes consciousness) as well as a balance of various elements within the body and foods eaten and balance of activities of daily living and spiritual pursuits. Ritual purity and cleanliness are also important for maintaining health. Because of the interrelatedness of mental and physical activity, a disturbance to one will cause a disturbance to the other. For example, fear, sadness, hurtfulness, or anger can contribute to sequelae like muscle tension, indigestion, or headache. The principles of balance are espoused in Ayurvedic theory, which recommends exercise, yoga, meditation, massage, steaming, and herbs as therapeutics.

Disease and disability are often also believed to result from karma (i.e., negative actions made in a past life) and are therefore resistant to treatment. Curses by a guru, elder, or accomplished one may also be believed by some to cause disease and epidemics. Being possessed by an evil spirit or demon is believed by some to cause death. Illness is framed as testing and a way to pay a past debt as well as an opportunity for learning and transformation (creating positive karma). Consequently, health-related decisions are not guided by what contributes to the best quantity or quality of life, but rather what fosters progress toward moksha. Healthcare decisions are also influenced by a variety of factors including: stage of life, gender, caste, timing (auspiciousness) of the diagnosis or treatment, perceived benefit for the good of others, and so forth. Thus:

- Hindus often hold negative attitudes toward use of pharmacologic agents to treat disease (e.g., antibiotics) and may think that Western healthcare providers overmedicate. Assessing how accepting of a possible prescription is merited.
- Ayurvedic approaches to healing may be used. Inform prescribing clinicians and/or pharmacists of any herbs being used. If not contraindicated and desired, facilitate or make a referral for hydrotherapy and/or massage.
- Be extra sensitive to the need for cleanliness, as Hindus are averse to becoming impure or dirty from bodily discharges. (See "Diet and Lifestyle: Prescriptions and Proscriptions.")
- When children experience a serious health challenge or deformity, the parents may suffer greatly, attributing it to their own or ancestral karma. Referral to a Hindu priest, or chaplain or counselor, may be helpful if wanted by the parents. Deep empathic listening can assist parents and other patients toward finding meaning and self-healing.
- Do not confuse acceptance of illness or suffering as fatalism or passivity; rather, they indicate spiritual development. Continue to provide education and treatment support.
- If mental healthcare is not holistic, a Hindu patient may not have confidence in it and be noncompliant. A soul or spirit does not exist independently from the mind or body. The adage "Adversity saves us from calamity" indicates how mental health is part of spiritual health.
- Support yogic practices (e.g., meditation, mantras, yoga) if requested. They may be perceived as more helpful than traditional Western therapeutics.

- Religious rituals (puja) requiring a priest may occur at a temple. If the patient cannot attend the puja, the priest will likely have the family take something tangible from the ceremony to the patient (e.g., temple food, a remnant of sacred cloth to be placed on the bed or worn around the shoulders). Show respect for such items.

Major health-related events often prompt need for a religious ritual (e.g., surgery or other significant procedures). Given the importance of purity, rituals symbolizing purification may also be performed after events like birthing, hospitalization, or mourning. Whereas these rituals usually occur at home, some (e.g., removal from life support) may occur in the hospital and need to be scheduled at an auspicious time (determined by the priest). Thus:

- If appropriate, inquire as to what clinical support is needed. Provide space and privacy for the ritual.

Beginning of Life: Beliefs and Practices

Incongruity between Hindu religious beliefs and Indian cultural practices is perhaps most evident when considering women's health and perinatal issues. Furthermore, practices may differ by the degree of Western influence on the patient. However, certain Hindu values influencing responses to beginning-of-life issues include the primacy of marriage, purity, nonviolence, and sacredness of all life. Several rituals are performed post partum or during infancy for the mother and/or child. Thus:

- Vaginal discharge (including menses) cause a woman to be impure, and they may avoid certain activities (e.g., touching others, intercourse, entering a temple), so they will avoid being close or touched by others during menses.
- Contraception that promotes family values and does not interfere with fertilization, alter body chemistry, or cause spotting may be preferred (e.g., abstinence, condoms).
- Although in India abortion has been prevalent for sex selection and population control, Hindu values such as nonviolence would dictate it only be used if needed to save the life of the mother. Indeed, the government of India has instituted programs for supporting the physical and mental health of pregnant women. However, in and outside of India, female feticide and infanticide do occur. This is often practiced against the woman's will, or with strong coercion. Sometimes the mother herself takes the action without others' knowledge.

- Likewise, it is believed that fetuses or infants with a defect (even if bad karma explains the defect) ought to be allowed to live their destiny, though magical remedies (incantations) may be invoked to placate the demon that may have caused the disease or deformity.

- Newly born may receive a tilaka (black mark) on the forehead for spiritual protection; there is no need to wash it away.

- It is not unusual for a mother to breastfeed a baby until it is 2 to 3 years old. If infant formula is used, teach the vegetarian mother to check formula ingredients, and ensure proper nutrition for both the mother and child.

- Prior to delivery, consult the mother regarding any ritual practices desired during hospitalization for child birthing and how nurses can best provide support (e.g., ceremonial washing of breasts prior to breastfeeding the infant the first time, or welcoming ceremony). Note that during the welcoming ceremony, honey or ghee (clarified butter) is placed on the baby's tongue; parents can be advised against use of honey for newborns less than 1 year old. Circumcision is never done.

- Given the higher value placed on male offspring (instead of female), there is often a marked difference in celebratory attitude after the birth of a daughter. This ought not to be misconstrued as postpartum depression.

End of Life: Beliefs and Practices

Death is the point of departure for the soul from the body. Given the soul is eternal and will pass on to a new life, death is not an enemy. The timing of one's death is determined by God. Death is defined as brain death (and for some, loss of body heat). Not only do beliefs about reincarnation and karma influence practices surrounding death, but they also influence values of ritual purity and compassion. Possibly the only time a priest will be called (i.e., hired) is when a death is imminent, because religious rituals are to be performed during and after a death. Thus:

- Hindus prefer to die at home. Family will be present and engaged in end-of-life decision making; extended family will likely be present at the time of death. Their crying will demonstrate their affection.

- Hindu women are not allowed to view a dead body. When a husband dies, the wife may not grieve his loss by being near his body. Likewise, the mother of a stillborn infant may refuse to hold her deceased child. Nurses should not misconstrue this as inappropriate coping; rather, it is the mother's (or her extended family's) religio-cultural expectations.

- Exactly when the death will occur is up to God; to provide a prognosis about timing is thought to invite premature dying. Thus, avoid talk about when the death is likely.

- Given God determines when death will occur, there is no need to prolong life artificially, as it will affect karma. Removal of hydration and food, however, is permissible. If a patient is to be removed from a ventilator and expected to die, a priest may be consulted to determine the correct time for doing so.

- Beliefs about karma as well as the desire for purity of body usually cause Hindus to reject organ transplantation (and sometimes blood transfusions); however, desiring longer life for spiritual development and compassion may counter antagonisms regarding organ donation and transplantation.

- Given the values of balance and keeping a clear mind, the patient in pain will likely want to titrate narcotics to balance pain and mental clarity. Yogic practices (e.g., mantras, hymn singing) will likely be comforting. Having a clear mind and remembering God at the time of death is thought to ensure moksha. Some may willfully choose to forgo analgesia, opting for a romanticized hero's death of intense suffering.

- Rituals that a priest and/or family may perform for the dying patient include reciting mantras and placing the patient's head in the direction where they perceive God exists.

- After the death, family may ritually bathe and enshroud the body (e.g., cover with oil or a paste, instill drops of holy water in the mouth). If a nurse is preparing the body, ask the family about removal of any marriage or religious pendants, strings, or jewelry.

- Unless necessary for legal or medical reasons, autopsies will not be desired. Embalming is not performed, and the body is cremated (unless it is that of a baby or very old person) within 24 hours. These practices are to facilitate the transition of the soul out of the body.

- During the mourning period of 10 to 40 days after the death, the family of the deceased may observe certain restrictions and rituals given their association with death puts them in an impure state.

Diet and Lifestyle: Prescriptions and Proscriptions

Hindus strive to keep the mind, body, and environment free from impurities. Thus:

- Support patients to bathe daily (morning preferred), and provide means for washing hands and mouth prior to meals and for washing hands after a meal. Promptly clean the body as needed after any "unclean" discharge (e.g., drooling, toileting, vomiting). Shoes may be removed prior to entering the home or hospital room.

- Know that historically the left hand was used for touching unclean things (e.g., excrement); therefore, it may be disturbing to hand a clean object (e.g., food, medication) to a patient using the left hand.

- To maintain a clear mind, narcotics are avoided unless necessary. Alcohol and caffeine are likewise avoided, although tea is a staple.

- Some Hindus are always vegetarian, while some may be vegetarian only during specified times. Traditional Hindus do not eat meat (especially pork and beef), fish, onions, garlic, salt, strong spices, eggs, commercial cheeses, and overripe fruit. Honey is preferred over sugar. They also seek to be moderate in the quantity of food consumed. The strict vegetarian may not want to take medications made with animal products (e.g., gelatin capsule).

Additional Miscellaneous Nursing Implications

- Do not expect a priest to visit; indeed, a priest may expect payment from the patient's family for a visit.

- Modesty is important to women; protect their modesty as much as possible during examinations and treatments. A nurse of the same gender may be preferred; if this is not possible, the presence of a family member may be invited.

- A patient may wear a talisman or symbol of marriage (e.g., string around the shoulder, gold pendant around the neck). Likewise, a married woman may wear a bindi, or red dot on the forehead. Respect and protect these symbols. If removal is necessary, ask permission, and consult as to how to keep worn objects safe.

- Given Indian collectivist culture, it is not unusual for elders to defer major healthcare decision making to their family (especially males).

Ways and Words to Comfort

- Ask how nurses can support religious (yogic) practices (see "Worship and Devotional Practices").

- Hindus will find comfort in remembering that no matter what happens to the body, the soul is unharmed. Indeed, suffering can allow one to reverse bad karma and generate good karma—and progress toward moksha. Use communication skills that allow a patient to take comfort in knowing this.

Bibliography

Dasa, S. (2012). Hindus. In E. J. Taylor (Ed.), *Religion: A clinical guide for nurses* (pp. 145–154). New York, NY: Springer Publishing.

Sharma, A. (2002). *The Hindu tradition: Religious beliefs and healthcare decisions.* Chicago, IL: Park Ridge Center. Retrieved from https://www.advocate health.com/assets/documents/faith/hindufinal.pdf

Simha, S., Noble, S., & Chaturvedi, S. K. (2013). Spiritual concerns in Hindu cancer patients undergoing palliative care: A qualitative study. *Indian Journal of Palliative Care, 19*(2), 99–105. doi:10.4103/0973-1075.116716

Singh, A., & Freeman, M. (2011). The important role for nurses in supporting the Asian Hindu patient and family at end of life: Providing culturally sensitive end-of-life care. *Canadian Oncology Nursing Journal, 21*(1), 46–49.

Srivastava, R., Srivastava, B., & Srivastava, R. (2011). Hinduism and nursing. In M. D. Fowler, S. Reimer-Kirkham, R. Sawatzky, & E. J. Taylor (Eds.), *Religion, religious ethics, and nursing* (pp. 173–196). New York, NY: Springer Publishing.

Sukumaran, A. (1999). *Hinduism and medicine.* Retrieved from http://www .angelfire.com/az/ambersukumaran/medicine.html

Tanenbaum Center for Interreligious Understanding. (2009). *The medical manual for religio-cultural competence* (pp. 108–122). New York, NY: Author.

23

Islam

Other Names and Similar Religious Traditions

Persons of the Islamic faith are Muslims. Whereas most Muslims are **Sunni**, smaller denominations include **Shia** and **Sufi**. Practices are similar among the denominations, but some differences in beliefs exist (e.g., about who should lead Muslims).

Social and Historical Background

Islam means submission to Allah (God). Islam began on the Arabian peninsula after God revealed to the most recent prophet, Muhammad (circa 570–632), the messages that now make up the holy book of the Qur'an (or Koran). Subsequently, further narration and explanation of the acts and sayings of Muhammad and his followers were recorded in Sunnah and hadiths.

Islam is not only a religion but a way of life. The abovementioned scriptures provide the Shari'a, the guidance about what is beneficial for mind and body, for living as families and societies, as well as for maintaining property and the environment. Shari'a encompasses five "pillars of faith" and provides the basis for beliefs. These include (1) confessing that there is no other God but Allah and that the prophet Muhammad is his messenger; (2) praying three (for Shia) or five (for Sunni) times a day; (3) paying 2.5% of one's income to charity if one has some savings; (4) fasting during Ramadan; and (5) making a pilgrimage to Mecca.

Worship and Devotional Practices

Weekly congregational ceremonial Islamic worship occurs at a mosque or Islamic cultural center every Friday at noon; whereas these are obligatory for men, women are welcome if family obligations do not make it burdensome. This service will include prayers and a sermon from the religious leader, an imam. Community-building activities and business will likely also occur.

More important than weekly religious service attendance, however, is fulfilling the obligation to perform formal salat prayers three or five times daily. These prayers are encouraged to be performed in congregation five times a day if possible by male Muslims in the mosque or at a convenient gathering place. These prayers must be preceded by ablutions. Those who cannot pray because of age or physical or mental illness are exempt, as are menstruating women. Patients unable to pray for a temporary reason are expected to make up their missed prayers. Muslims also may recite prayers for any number of things throughout the day (e.g., before eating, leaving one's house). To not pray is sinful. Thus:

- Formal prayers involve assuming various positions (standing, kneeling, bending, prostration). For the patient who is unable to move well, prayers can be said while sitting (with chest facing Mecca, Saudi Arabia—where Muhammad was born) or lying in bed (with feet facing Mecca), or even by thinking through or imaging the movements. Some patients will use their eye movements in place of bodily movements. Many Muslims have a smartphone application that provides a compass to determine the direction in which to pray.
- Ablutions (*wudhu*) involve thoroughly washing one's face (including mouth, nose, and ears), hands, forearms, and hair. Thus, bring a pan of clean water to the patient if needed; if unable to have water at the bedside, a pan with sand can substitute.
- Formal prayers (salat) are recited during specified intervals that are based on the position of the sun; thus, the time varies with season and geographical location. Very simply, these prayers occur at dawn, midday, late afternoon, just after sunset, and late evening.
- Once begun, a Muslim will not interrupt the prayer—not even for a crying child or for a nurse.

All prayers are recitations from the holy book, Qur'an. Islam is an oral tradition, and all Muslims memorize portions of the Qur'an. Many Muslims memorize the entire Qur'an. Because it is a holy book, it is to be treated with utmost respect.

- Ablutions are necessary prior to touching the Qur'an. The non-Muslim nurse should either not touch the Qur'an or wrap it in a clean cloth if needing to handle it. Never place a Qur'an on the floor, and never place anything on top of it.

- Many Muslims have smartphone applications for listening to Quranic recitations in Arabic, which may be selected with or without translation into other languages.

Another worshipful obligation is the fast of Ramadan, which is celebrated during the month when Muhammad received the first revelations that comprise the Qur'an. Ramadan varies from year to year, given a lunar calendar is followed. The fast involves abstaining from all food, drink, and intermarital relations between dawn and sunset during these 29 to 30 days. In addition to fasting, Muslims seek forgiveness, practice charity, and observe religious devotional practices (e.g., reading the entire Qur'an) to draw closer to Allah. Exempt from the fast are the seriously ill (including diabetics); elderly; pregnant, lactating, or menstruating women; and prepubescent children. Those exempted, if able, are to later make up the fast or take food to the poor. Thus, during Ramadan:

- Those who need oral or other medication should not fast. For those who insist on fasting, however, adjust oral or injectable medications and intravenous fluids to be delivered during the night (after sundown and before dawn). Because these would contain nutrients, receiving them would negate the fast.
- Permitted therapeutics include eye or ear drops, dental care, inhalers, nebulizer treatments, nasal sprays, immunizations, and insulin injections.
- If a medication is essential during the daytime fast to improve health, it should be administered regardless of route.
- Even though they are exempt, some patients may try to observe Ramadan to experience solidarity with fellow Muslims.
- Predawn and postevening meals should include foods with low glycemic index, or carbohydrates that release energy slowly (e.g., steel-cut oats, sweet potatoes, nonstarchy vegetables, nuts).
- If patients with diabetes mellitus want to fast, negotiate with them to refrain from fully observing the fast, or recommend that they monitor their blood sugar and take a supplement or end the fast if they experience hypoglycemia.

Muslims who are physically and financially able are to fulfill the obligation at least once during their lifetime to make a pilgrimage to Mecca, Saudi Arabia (where Muhammad was born and received the Quranic revelations). The hajj pilgrimage is made during a specified 5- to 6-day period, whereas the *Umrah* pilgrimage is shorter and can be done at any time. (Muslims who are not performing hajj may also fast.) Both involve several rituals and considerable walking. Thus, for those preparing for this pilgrimage:

- Provide information and resources to address the potential health problems that can arise from prolonged exposure to millions of people and miles of walking in the desert environment (e.g., dehydration and heat-related conditions, respiratory and gastrointestinal and other communicable diseases, foot care). For example, prophylactic antibiotics, sturdy and padded footwear, and so forth can be advised. (Note that there are restrictions for men on types of footwear worn during certain days in hajj.) The World Health Organization (WHO), Centers for Disease Control and Prevention (CDC), and Saudi Arabian Ministry of Health provide preparatory heath information for hajj pilgrims.
- The Saudi Arabian Ministry of Health annually updates medical requirements for those requesting a travel visa for the hajj or Umrah; vaccination requirements vary by country of travel origin. Visit www.moh.gov.sa/en/hajj/pages/healthregulations.aspx.
- Because of a belief that death while performing hajj earns one a heavenly reward, some on this pilgrimage may neglect caring for their chronic illnesses. Although Saudi Arabia offers free healthcare to pilgrims who become ill or injured, many such visits could be avoided if pilgrims simply continued their current medications. Urge pilgrims to continue to take their medications or treatments for any current chronic diseases during the hajj.

Illness and Healing: Beliefs and Practices

Muslims view health as a blessing from Allah that ought not to be misused. Health is defined holistically and involves balancing mind, body, and soul; indeed, having a strong relationship with Allah promotes health, and faith is requisite to healing. The Islamic scriptures provide holistic guidelines for what to do to be well. For example, one is to choose good instead of evil, balance personal with collective needs, and maintain cleanliness. Thus, when a Muslim becomes sick, it is common for that person to spend more time in prayer and devotion to God (e.g., to seek forgiveness, read or listen to the Qur'an, give more to charity, eat and drink certain foods) as well as to seek a scientific cure.

Although the Muslim will seek healing, they will also find comfort in certain beliefs about illness and tragedy. For instance, Allah knows the destiny of all persons, and nothing happens without His permission. How persons respond to trials reflects their free will;

thus, Muslims will pray to face adversity with patience and thereby receive expiation for their sins. Thus:

- Families and imams may recite specific chapters of the Qur'an in the presence of the patient. Not only do Muslims pray for those who are sick, there is also importance placed on the prayers of the sick for others.

Muslims may use a traditional therapeutic referenced in the Qur'an or Hadith. These include eating or topically applying honey or taking dates, herbs, olives, (camel) milk, aloe, capers, chicory, black cumin, dill, fenugreek, pomegranate, indigo, senna, mustard, truffles, *Nigella sativa*, or zam zam water (holy water from Mecca). Thus:

- When caring for those disorders such as depression, schizophrenia, and other mental health challenges, talk about these illnesses as having a physiological component. With this framing, they will be more accepting of antidepressants and other medications.

Beginning of Life: Beliefs and Practices

A soul is believed to enter a fetus at the end of the 4th month of pregnancy (120 days). Islam places much value on family life; Muslims enjoy having children and raise close-knit families. It is usual for young adults to live at home until they marry. Premarital and extramarital affairs are forbidden. Thus:

- Postcoital contraception and sterilization are unacceptable.
- Treatment for fertility is encouraged, if it does not involve a donor (as that would be akin to adultery) or disrupt lineage.
- Abortion is prohibited except in cases of incest, rape, or if the mother's life is threatened.

In conservative Middle Eastern Islamic cultures, tension exists regarding open discussion of sexuality. This may contribute to a lack of knowledge and misperceptions about some women's health issues. For example, universal offering of human papillomavirus vaccination is thought to deter chastity among youth and is one barrier to its delivery to young women (Hamdi, 2018). Thus:

- Provide sexual health information, as it may be meager for Muslim women from conservative Islamic societies. Provide it, however, with sensitivity for conservative sexual mores.
- Have a nurse of the same gender provide any reproductive health care and information. Be sensitive to the reality that a Muslim

immigrant woman may have great difficulty talking about sexuality.

■ Although gynecological examinations are common for married or previously married women, single Muslim women may refuse such an exam for fear of compromising her virginity.

When a Muslim mother delivers a child, she is to recite specific prayers. Once the infant is born, the father, a relative, or imam is to recite a call to prayer into the ears of the infant. Male circumcision is obligatory and may be performed at different possible times prior to age 7. Female genital mutilation is not described in any of the Islamic holy books.

End of Life: Beliefs and Practices

Death is viewed as the entry to the next life. At death, the spirit sleeps until the Day of Judgment. The reward of bliss (paradise) or devastation (hell) will be based on one's faith and actions during life. (Allah/God, however, is most merciful and compassionate when one seeks forgiveness after failing one of life's many trials.) Allah has complete authority over human's destiny. This means that although people are to seek a cure, they must not unnecessarily "play God" and try to control or prolong life. Thus:

■ Muslims often pray for forgiveness and admission to paradise, to be with loved ones, the prophets, and God.
■ The belief in an eternal afterlife in paradise brings comfort to the dying.
■ Remind those who fear the Day of Judgment because of their sins that God is all-forgiving and all-merciful.
■ Euthanasia and assisted suicide are forbidden.

Because only Allah knows the time for death, Muslims avoid speaking about a loved one's death until it is upon them. Death and burial practices include the following:

■ When death is imminent, patients (or family proxy) are encouraged to confess their faith (i.e., "There is no God except Allah, and Muhammad is his prophet"), repent, and anticipate Allah's mercy. Any passage from the Qur'an is also read. Thus, Muslims prefer pain management that does not interfere with the ability to pray at the moment just before death. Muslims will take pain medication, especially if it is recommended by their physician.
■ After the death, the body is ritually cleansed by family or Muslim community members of the same gender as the deceased as well

as a trusted Muslim who knows the ritual. The body is anointed and enshrouded in three white sheets (for men) and sheets plus clothing (for women).

- Cremation, embalming, and autopsies (unless legally or medically necessary) are forbidden.
- The body will be taken immediately to the mosque where prayers for the deceased are said (within 72 hours of death). Then the funeral will occur at the cemetery. Because men want to protect women from the raw emotion of watching a casket-less burial, women are discouraged from attending, but they may do so.
- Burial within 1 day of the death is preferred; however, it may be delayed to allow close family to come to attend.
- Given the short time frame from death to burial, a death certificate should be signed quickly.

Islamic tradition also guides mourning practices. Depending on denomination, certain memorial days are set aside (3rd, 7th, or 40th day after death anniversary). A widow is to mourn at least 4 months and 10 days and may not even leave her house.

Consultative support for Muslims addressing ethical dilemmas can be found at Islamic Medical Association of North America (imana.org). This site offers a 24/7 hotline for questions about palliative care concerns. For example, while organ donation is generally acceptable, it does vary depending on the circumstances.

Diet and Lifestyle: Prescriptions and Proscriptions

Permissible (halal) food excludes meat that has significant traces of blood, that has not been slaughtered properly (i.e., according to Islamic customs, in the name of Allah), or that comes from pork or any animal with claws. Muslims also recommend eating in moderation. Most will abstain from alcohol and not smoke or use illicit drugs. Thus:

- Avoid medications containing alcohol or porcine by-products (e.g., gelatin, syrups with alcohol).
- If a halal meal is not available, a Jewish kosher meal or vegetarian meal will suffice.

Additional Miscellaneous Nursing Implications

- Incorporating Islamic beliefs into patient education may improve adherence (e.g., Kamoun & Spatz, 2018).
- Sometimes, Muslims make ablution (wudhu) not just before prayer or handling the Qur'an but also when sick. It cleanses the

patient from the distractions of life and enhances communication with Allah.

■ Remember that healthcare decisions are made collectively by the family (vs. by the individual patient). Furthermore, male family members usually hold the authority to make decisions for the women in the family.

■ Because Islamic teachings include an obligation to visit the sick, patients will often have many visitors. Nurses may need to make accommodations or discuss limitations.

■ Imams, the clergy for Muslims, are typically available to visit a patient by arrangement. They are appropriate resources for spiritual comfort and religious wisdom.

■ In communities where there are many Muslims, there will be an Islamic Community Center/Society/Association with a mosque. Included in their offerings are often resources and services for the sick and elders.

■ Respecting the modesty of Muslim men and women is paramount. Details about how to respect the need for modesty include:
  ■ Offer nurses of the same gender to attend; offer fellow Muslims, if possible.
  ■ Depending on culture, to be fully covered can mean having all but face and hands exposed (for women) and the area between the navel and knees kept covered (for men).
  ■ Discourse between a man and woman not married to each other ought to be limited to only to what is necessary for professional or educational reasons.
  ■ Allow women to wear a head cover (if desired); allow time for them to place this on their head before entering their room.

Ways and Words to Comfort

■ "*In sha Allah*" (meaning "by God's will") is a phrase commonly interjected in Muslim discourse. Some Islamic hospitals have the motto "We care, but Allah heals." Restating or paraphrasing such ideas will comfort.

■ A Hadith admonishes believers to "keep the tongue moist" by repeating the name of Allah. A patient can repeat a short phrase or prayer silently or out loud as a form of meditation and remembrance of Allah.

■ Listening to the Qur'an is healing. The patient's family may do the reading, or a smartphone application with the reading of the Qur'an can be played.

■ Because the virtue of patience in times of illness or adversity is the correct response denoting trust in God, the nurse can validate for this virtue when it manifests in the patient.

- For immigrant Muslims who may think a board-certified chaplain (BCC) is a proselytizer, the nurse can explain how BCCs are trained to provide spiritual care across religions. If the patient is receptive, the nurse can formally introduce the chaplain to the patient, per social custom of many Islamic cultures. Of course, if available, refer to a Muslim chaplain.

Bibliography

Ali, M. (2012). Muslims. In E. J. Taylor (Ed.), *Religion: A clinical guide for nurses* (pp. 213–220). New York, NY: Springer Publishing.

Attum, B., & Shamoon, Z. (2018). *Cultural competence in the care of Muslim patients and their families.* Treasure Island, FL: StatPearls Publishing. Retrieved from https://www.ncbi.nlm.nih.gov/books/NBK499933

Hamdi, S. (2018). The impact of teachings on sexuality in Islam on HPV vaccine acceptability in the Middle East and North Africa region. *Journal of Epidemiology & Global Health, 7*(Suppl. 1), S17–S22. doi:10.1016/j.jegh.2018.02.003

Kamoun, C., & Spatz, D. (2018). Influence of Islamic traditions on breastfeeding beliefs and practices among African American Muslims in West Philadelphia: A mixed-methods study. *Journal of Human Lactation, 34*(1), 164–175. doi:10.1177/0890334417705856

Mujallad, A., & Taylor, E. J. (2016). Modesty among Muslim women: Implications for nursing care. *MEDSURG Nursing, 25*(3), 169–172.

Shafi, S., Dar, O., Khan, M., Khan, M., Azhar, E. I., McCloskey, B., . . . Petersen, E. (2016). The annual Hajj pilgrimage—minimizing the risk of ill health in pilgrims from Europe and opportunity for driving the best prevention and health promotion guidelines. *International Journal of Infectious Diseases, 47,* 79–82. doi:10.1016/j.ijid.2016.06.013

Waugh, E. H. (1999). *The Islamic tradition: Religious beliefs and healthcare decisions.* Chicago, IL: Park Ridge Center. Retrieved from https://www.advocatehealth.com/assets/documents/faith/islamic_tradition.pdf

24

Judaism: Conservative

Other Names and Similar Religious Traditions

Other names include **Masorti Judaism**, or **Masorti International** (see also Chapters 25 and 26).

Social and Historical Background

Judaism traces its roots to Abraham (c. 1700 BCE). The Halacha (the collective religious law, based on the Hebrew Bible and various subsequent rabbinic interpretations and amplifications) is central to Conservative Jewish life; it is to be obeyed yet applied in ways that are responsive to contemporary society. Indeed, this tension between obeying an historical law and adjusting religious practices to accommodate living in contemporary society is what distinguishes it from Orthodox Judaism. The Conservative Jewish denomination, a moderate movement (between Orthodox and liberal Jewish movements), was formalized in the mid-1900s. Its adherents, however, are rarely strictly observant of Jewish religious practices.

Worship and Devotional Practices

Jews communicate with God by praying, by studying, by practicing God's laws as interpreted in the tradition, and by improving the lives of others (i.e., *Tikkun Olam*, or repairing the world). Prayers are recited (memorized or read from a prayer book) daily in the morning, afternoon, and evening, as well as a blessing before and after a meal (see Chapter 25 for more detail). Prayer can also be meditative or spontaneously formed to communicate with God. Whereas prayer can occur at any place, prayer in the context of a minyan (quorum of 10) is preferred. Thus:

- Provide uninterrupted quiet time—especially in the morning.
- Assist patients to don a *kippah* (skullcap or head covering), a sign of respect for God, worn during worship if not all day.

Sabbath/Shabbat, a holy day for rejuvenation, is celebrated every Saturday, from dusk Friday to when "three stars" can be seen in the evening sky of Saturday. In addition to attending synagogue services (Friday after sundown, Sabbath morning, and before sundown on Sabbath), the 24-hour period is to include three sumptuous meals. To avoid work on Sabbath, therefore, preparations are made on Friday (i.e., meals cooked, home cleaned, clothing in order). Sabbath afternoon activities can include visiting with fellow believers after a wonderful meal, walking, sleeping, and reading (e.g., holy scripture). All work is to be avoided (e.g., lighting a fire—interpreted today as starting a car or using electricity to open a door or light a room [see Chapter 25]). Five major and several minor festivals are celebrated by Jews. They are celebrated much like a Sabbath but will have other unique attributes. The degree to which a Conservative Jew observes these practices reflects the degree of their orthodoxy. Thus:

- Prior to Friday evening, discuss with the patient/family how they would want to celebrate Sabbath, likewise, major Jewish holy days (e.g., provide apple dipped in honey for Rosh Hashanah, symbolic of hope for a sweet new year).
- Nonurgent or necessary care may be refused on Sabbath or holy days.
- If possible, coparticipate in a brief ritual to start Shabbat (i.e., have the patient "light" two battery-operated candles, provide a roll of bread [preferably an egg bread] and taste of wine/grape juice to be blessed); alternatively, turn the room lights off prior to sundown, and then intentionally turn them on at sundown with an acknowledgment of this blessed time (e.g., "Shabbat shalom" or "Peace!").

Illness and Healing: Beliefs and Practices

Saving life overrides all other values. For example, if a blood transfusion will save a life, it is acceptable even though kosher law restricts consuming blood. Jews believe that they have a sacred duty to take care of health because the body belongs to God, as does everything else. Jews are to take care of their health to the extent that they can (e.g., avoid excessive alcohol, smoking, and opt for health-promoting behaviors), but they should also realize that many diseases just happen, regardless of one's health behaviors, morality, or piety. Jews ascribe meaning to suffering in two ways. First, suffering allows one to gain wisdom; second, it allows the community to rally to care for the sufferer. Thus:

- Health promotion strategies can include recognizing this sacred duty to preserve the body belonging to God.
- Although it is important to allow patients to process how they make sense of serious illness and disability, these Jewish attributions (i.e., suffering allows wisdom and strengthens community) may resonate with the Jewish patient.

Beginning of Life: Beliefs and Practices

Conservative and Orthodox Jews accept the command to procreate and take a biblical story to mean that noncoital sexual acts are immoral and that a man's semen is not to be emitted without purpose. While some interpret this to mean contraception is not permissible, some Conservative Jews will condone an intrauterine device, an oral contraceptive, spermicide, or diaphragm. Given there is more intermarrying among Conservative Jews, the rates for genetic diseases and anomalies are presumably less (compared to Orthodox Jews, Chapter 25). Thus:

- Confirm what method of birth control, if any, are permissible to a patient.

Other considerations while caring for infants include:

- Infant boys will be circumcised on the 8th day of life; given there is no equivalent ceremony for girls, some parents may create one (e.g., pour water over the feet). Infants will be named in a naming ceremony at home or a synagogue.
- Use kosher (e.g., soy) formula for babies requiring supplemental feeding.

End of Life: Beliefs and Practices

Orthodox and Conservative Jews do not cremate. They believe the dead are "gathered to their ancestors" (Judges 2:9); this biblical text suggests there is an afterlife that involves reconnection with one's deceased family. Organ donation is encouraged. Several customs are practiced to honor the deceased and to appreciate how death equalizes all persons. These customs include burial as soon as possible within 24 hours (or 48 hours, if it is Sabbath or a holy day, or immediate family are unable to come sooner); burial in a simple pine box; washing and dressing the body in a simple white shroud; and never leaving the deceased's body until it is buried. Mourning practices allow family and friends to provide intense social support to the bereaved. Family will "sit shiva" for 3 (for the less conservative) to 7 days (for the more conservative and Orthodox Jews). Supporters will bring food and reminisce and function to create a minyan for prayers; flowers are not appropriate. Thus:

- When death is imminent, support the patient's family to contact the local synagogue to make arrangements (e.g., determine if there is a burial society that will come and wash and dress the body after the death; if not, family members of the same gender as deceased may want to use warm water to wash their loved one's body, being mindful to never let it face downward, and enshroud it).
- There are prayers that Jews recite when death is near. These include a prayer accepting God's justice and a confessional asking for forgiveness.
- Once the patient has died, close the eyelids.
- Accommodate any family member who will insist on remaining with the body.
- If visiting the family sitting *shiva* after the death, one can bring food (kosher food, if the family keeps kosher) or do other things to support the daily lives of the bereaved.

Diet and Lifestyle: Prescriptions and Proscriptions

Many Conservative and all Orthodox Jews eat kosher ("correct") food. Kosher dictates include eating only meat from cloven-hoofed animals, only fish with scales and fins, and no insects or birds of prey. Any animal-based food must be slaughtered in a humane way by a trained Jewish butcher. Given no blood is to be eaten, meat is salted to remove blood. Meat and dairy are not to be eaten together or within a specified length of time of each other. Given this rule, many Jews keep two separate sets of dishes to not risk mixing meat and dairy. Holy days often require feasting (e.g., during Passover, symbolic foods including nonleavened foods are eaten) or fasting (i.e., Yom Kippur). Thus:

- Avoid foods (e.g., gelatin, lard or shortening, glycerin, rennet in cheeses) or medications (nonvegetarian gel capsules and chewables) that contain derivatives of non-kosher foods.
- If unsure, serve only food labeled with the kosher logo, fresh fruits or vegetables, or a prepackaged kosher meal (which should remain sealed while heating, and not be unsealed until in the presence of the patient; serve with disposable dinnerware).

- If vegetarian medications and kosher food are not available, yet necessary to support life, then it is acceptable. Likewise, if a fast is deleterious to health, it is not to be observed.

Additional Miscellaneous Nursing Implications

- More traditional Jews will want to wash their hands thrice, using a cup, upon waking as well as before meals.
- Some Jews, especially older ones or those from the Orient, may be superstitious and observe some different practices. A common one is to tie a red ribbon around the bedpost to ward off evil spirits. Another is to put one of the psalms on the headboard to invoke the presence of God.
- *Bikkur Holim* (congregation-based groups tasked to visit the sick in institutions or at home) and Jewish Family Services (community-based organizations that provide in-home social services like transportation and meal preparation) are resources.

Ways and Words to Comfort

See Chapter 26 regarding ways to support prayer.

Bibliography

Chabad. (n.d.). *Jewish practice.* Retrieved from https://www.chabad.org/library/article_cdo/aid/1675888/jewish/Jewish-Practice.htm

Hoffman, L. (2018). A focus on: Judaism. *Community Practitioner, 91*(2), 31–33.

The Jewish Federation of Greater Washington. (2019). *Jewish traditions explained.* Retrieved from https://www.jconnect.org/Resources/Jewish-Traditions-Explained

Jewish Visiting. (n.d.). *Caring for a Jewish patient: A guide for medical professionals.* Retrieved from https://jvisit.org.uk/caring-for-a-jewish-patient-a-guide-for-medical-professionals

Jotkowitz, A. B., Clarfield, A. M., & Glick, S. (2005). The care of patients with dementia: A modern Jewish ethical perspective. *Journal of the American Geriatrics Society, 53*(5), 881–884. doi:10.1111/j.1532-5415.2005.53271.x

25

Judaism: Orthodox

Other Names and Similar Religious Traditions

At the most conservative end of the Jewish spectrum are the **Orthodox Jews** (see also Chapters 24 and 26 on Conservative and Reform Judaism). Those who integrate themselves into secular culture are **Modern Orthodox** or **Religious Zionists**; Orthodox Jews who view contemporary culture as a threat and insulate themselves from secular society are **Haredi(m)**, or **Ultra-Orthodox** (considered by some a pejorative label). Although there are many subgroups of Haredim, **Hasidic** and **Lithuanian Yeshivish** (**Litvaks**) are most common.

Social and Historical Background

Orthodox Jews perceive they are the most authentic continuance of ancient Judaism. They developed in the 1700s as a reformation response to liberalizing movements within Judaism. Today, it is estimated there may be 500,000 Orthodox Jews in the United States; a concentration of about 340,000 Ultra-Orthodox Jews live around New York City.

Long-standing Jewish traditions are maintained among Orthodox Jews; indeed, religion dominates the way of life. The Halacha (Hebrew scriptures and rabbinic teachings) provides the law by which adherents live their lives, and rabbis provide guidance on how to apply these laws. They live in patriarchal and large families. Religious training is of greatest importance and begins at a young age for boys. There is variation, however, in how much secular education is obtained among Orthodox Jews. While some are highly educated and work in professional roles, others may not have a college degree. Indeed, substantial variations in how Modern or Zionist Orthodox and the more conservative Haredim relate to healthcare will reflect the underlying difference of belief about how to integrate into secular society.

Worship and Devotional Practices

Shabbat (Sabbath), observed from sundown Friday to 1 hour past sundown on Saturday, is a time of rest from work and for communal celebration with the synagogue congregation and family. Thus, there is no use of electricity (or anything involving the lighting of a spark), no bathing, no exchange of money, no writing, no phoning, and so forth. Thus:

- Recognize that hospitalized Jewish patients may be particularly lonely on Shabbat if their family members are unable to walk the distance to visit them.
- Bring two electric candles at the start of Shabbat to women, who traditionally light these symbols of holy time.
- Before Shabbat, plan with the patient for appropriate garments and food for this special day.
- Avoid discharge on Shabbat.
- Do not expect the patient to push a button (e.g., nurse call light), pass through an electric door, sign a consent form, and so forth, on Shabbat. Turn on lights and machinery prior to Shabbat; discuss with the patient/family other implications of Shabbat observance before it begins.

Men pray thrice a day (expectations for women are less and vary by subgroup): 20 to 40 minutes within 2 hours of daylight and 5 to 10 minutes both in the afternoon and evening (often at nightfall and sometimes back to back with the afternoon prayers). Prayers include established blessings, Psalms, and other scriptural passages. Men will wear a prayer shawl and *keffelin* (small black boxes with Scripture inside, which are strapped to the forehead and upper arm during prayers). Most recite prayers while standing, swaying, and facing east (toward the holy city of Jerusalem). Individual prayer is good; group prayer is better (in a minyan of at least 10 men who have celebrated their religious initiation [bar mitzvah] at age 13). Thus:

- Support male patients with positioning and accoutrements for prayer in the morning and afternoon/evening, as requested.
- Facilitate space for large group (minyan) who may come to pray for a patient.
- Plan daily schedule to allow for the three prayer services.

Illness and Healing: Beliefs and Practices

Preserving and saving life is a fundamental value; this does not necessarily mean, however, prolonging suffering. The dignity of a person must be maintained, and it is laudable to provide care. Explanations for illness can vary and be multilayered (e.g., divine will, biology). Thus:

- Medication for managing pain and other symptoms will be accepted.
- Treatments are not to be withdrawn unless the patient improves; alternatively, if an "intermittent treatment" was initiated, then during a pause in this treatment plan, it can be determined that it is best to discontinue or change the plan—often per the counsel of the rabbi.
- Causal attributions will influence responses to illness.

Rabbis (called *posek*, the *Rebbe*, or the *Rov*) are conduits of God to humans; all major life decisions are made in consultation with these men. Their word will carry more weight than those of a judge or physician. Thus:

- Patients/families will frequently consult their rabbi about significant healthcare decisions (e.g., contraception, surgery or other major treatments, end-of-life decisions).
- More than one rabbi may be consulted; each could provide a different recommendation.
- Facilitate inclusion of rabbis in decision making, as desired by the patient/family.

Beginning of Life: Beliefs and Practices

Given the imperative to "be fruitful and multiple," birth rates are very high (on average around seven children per woman). Women marry young and view pregnancy as a way of life, a way of enacting their piety. Given the consanguineous communities, the rates for some genetically based diseases and birth anomalies are high (e.g., *BRCA* gene, cystic fibrosis). Pregnancy and the condition of the fetus are God's choice; if the fetus is abnormal, that is interpreted as a test of faith, and possibly an affirmation of God's confidence in the mother. Thus:

- Contraception is prohibited unless necessary for the well-being of the woman; the form of contraception will be recommended by the rabbi.
- Prenatal testing is a spiritual ordeal, and it is often refused; rabbinic council is often sought and may change the parents' decision.
- Pregnant women may reject a test by simply saying something like, "We don't do that"; sensitive inquiry about what prompts this response will be helpful.

- An international genetic testing program, Dor Yeshorim (doryeshorim.org), provides free premarital testing to any Jew and information for Jewish families of children with genetic diseases.
- Jewish organizations exist to support Jewish children with such special needs.

Sexuality is sacred, and a husband is not to touch his wife while she is menstruating or discharging lochia. Thus:

- A husband is not to have sex with his wife during and up to 1 week after menstruation (or spotting), when she has the ritual bath (mikveh) at the synagogue.
- Once labor begins, a husband will not touch his wife; during the delivery, he is not to view the actual birthing but may stand at the head of her bed or behind a screen.

Early life events for an infant include circumcision (for males) and a naming ceremony. Thus:

- Accommodate completion of a birth certificate until after the naming.
- Infant boys will be circumcised on the eighth day of life (or when the infant is well enough) by a trained Jewish circumciser in the synagogue or home.

End of Life: Beliefs and Practices

Suffering is not seen as redemptive and should be alleviated. The tradition recognizes different stages of end of life. Thus:

- Rabbinic guidance can vary depending on the end-of-life stage of the patient.
- Opioids and pain management are appropriate, but not euthanasia.
- Advance directives or Physician Orders for Life-Sustaining Treatment (POLST) are acceptable.
- A home environment is preferred; if not feasible, bringing items from home to the healthcare setting can help to create a feeling of home.

Multiple European pogroms to eradicate Jews during the past 150 years also continue to color the orthodox Jews' reality. Thus,

- Use of hydration or parenteral nutrition (thought to be akin to hand feeding) may be chosen from a preconscious fear of starvation.

Burial and mourning practices are akin to those practiced by Conservative Jews (see Chapter 24).

Diet and Lifestyle: Prescriptions and Proscriptions

Orthodox Jews will be particularly observant of kosher laws (see Chapter 24 for information). Thus:

- Confirm kosher diet with dietary department; check with the patient whether members of family or *Bikur Holim* will bring any food, and inform them of any dietary orders.

Additional Miscellaneous Nursing Implications

Sexuality is very private; modesty is important. In public, married women wear dresses that cover elbows and knees and head covering (usually a hat, scarf, and/or wig). Men and women are to have limited interaction and avoid casual conversation. Thus:

- When entering the patient's room, knock and give a moment for women to cover themselves.
- Women may want to wear a head covering (e.g., surgical cap) and use extra gowns or blankets for covering.
- Avoid handshakes, hugs, or touch with Ultra-Orthodox Jews of the opposite gender.
- If alone with a patient of the opposite gender, understand this can cause anxiety; leave the door ajar, or invite another person of the opposite gender to be present.

Ultra-Orthodox Jews primarily speak Yiddish (English is commonly a second language), and communities are tight-knit with marriages arranged to couple those with disabilities or other stigmatized health challenges. Thus:

- A patient with a mental health or other stigmatized condition may be loath to have a Yiddish translator present; use off-site translation services (e.g., telephone), if preferred.
- Potentially stigmatized patients (or their parents) may take considerable effort to ensure privacy—even within the family.
- When receiving healthcare, Orthodox Jewish patients may be exposed to television and other aspects of a secular society for the first time and may be anxious or overwhelmed.
- Patients may fear their beliefs and practices will be undermined or disrespected by non-Jewish clinicians.

Families are large; extended family likely live close. Thus:

- Make space or negotiate how family can be present for patients.
- Identify a direct line of communication between a family representative and clinicians.

Words and Ways to Comfort

See Chapter 26 regarding ways to support prayer.

Bibliography

Bressler, T., & Popp, B. (2018). Ethical challenges when caring for Orthodox Jewish patients at the end of life. *Journal of Hospice and Palliative Care Nursing, 20*(1), 36–44. doi:10.1097/NJH.0000000000000402

Gabbay, E., McCarthy, M., & Fins, J. (2017). The care of the Ultra-Orthodox Jewish patient. *Journal of Religion & Health, 56*(2), 545–560. doi:10.1007/s10943-017-0356-6

Ivry, T., Teman, E., & Frumkin, A. (2011). God-sent ordeals and their discontents: Ultra-orthodox Jewish women negotiate prenatal testing. *Social Science & Medicine, 72*(9), 1527–1533. doi:10.1016/j.socscimed.2011.03.007

Popovsky, M. A. (2010). Special issues in the care of Ultra-Orthodox Jewish psychiatric in-patients. *Transcultural Psychiatry, 47*(4), 647–672. doi:10.1177/1363461510383747

Semenic, S. E., Callister, L. C., & Feldman, P. (2004). Giving birth: The voices of Orthodox Jewish women living in Canada. *Journal of Obstetric, Gynecologic & Neonatal Nursing, 33*(1), 80–87. doi:10.1177/0884217503258352

26

Judaism: Reform

Other Names and Similar Religious Traditions

In contrast to Orthodox and Conservative Judaism, the **Reform** (or **Liberal** or **Progressive Judaism**) and **Reconstructionist** denominations accept that Judaism must adapt to contemporary culture. The **Alliance for Jewish Renewal** (aleph.org/what-is-jewish-renewal) is a socially progressive, transdenominational Jewish organization with aims that include enlivening Jews' spiritual experience by learning from Hasidism and mystical Jewish traditions (e.g., Kabbalah).

Social and Historical Background

Although Judaism is one of the world's oldest religions, in modern times its adherents have varied in their interpretations of what it means to believe and belong. Both these liberal movements were formalized in the United States in the 1900s. These denominations are socially progressive; they are inclusive of homosexual/transgendered persons, treat women with equality, accept intermarriage between a Jew and non-Jew, and reject that a Jew is defined as born to a Jewish woman. In Reform Judaism, decision making about how to interpret and apply Jewish law (Halacha) is done jointly by rabbis and lay members. In Reconstructionist Judaism, the congregations determine how to practice Judaism, but this is not based on a belief that the Halacha is religious law (rather, it is "folkways"). Although over the recent few decades Reform Jews have readopted many traditional practices, many adherents see religious behaviors as optional and a personal choice. Given the liberal persuasion, there is an acceptance of diverse religious beliefs and practices in these denominations.

Worship and Devotional Practices

In these denominations, many traditional Jewish practices are no longer observed, or they are retained (sometimes adapted). Thus, some Reform Jews attend synagogue on Sunday, rather than Sabbath. Dietary and hygienic prescriptions may not be practiced. Thus:

- Assess what religious practices do impact healthcare (e.g., "For what diet, hygiene, or religious rituals will you need support?")
- Reconstructionists and Reform have their own prayer books. Like more conservative Jews, they may pray in Hebrew thrice daily or in their own vernacular.
- Many will still observe Sabbath from Friday sundown to Saturday sundown with the traditional meals and synagogue attendance. A Reform Jewish website offers online Sabbath prayers and streaming of synagogue services (reformjudaism.org/jewish-holidays/shabbat).

Illness and Healing: Beliefs and Practices

Whereas the rabbi is integrally involved and directive for orthodox Jews making significant healthcare decisions, the culture of liberal Jewish denominations heavily involves laity in the process of applying religious law. Therefore, liberal Jewish patients may be less inclined to consult a rabbi.

Beginning of Life: Beliefs and Practices

Liberal Jews do practice circumcision, as it represents the covenantal relationship to Jewish people. Contraceptives (including diaphragm) are permissible. Abortion under certain circumstances is supported, especially if it is within 40 days of conception or pregnancy threatens the mother's life.

End of Life: Beliefs and Practices

Jewish law is thought to offer resources, not absolutes, on how to make end-of-life decisions. Although end-of-life beliefs and practices described in Chapters 24 and 25 are pertinent, there likely will be less strict adherence to traditional Jewish practices of burying the dead. For example, Reform Jews do allow embalming; they also approve of cremation. It also may be that they "sit shiva" for only 3 days. Organ donation is encouraged. Some liberal Jews may not believe in an afterlife. Thus:

- An attempt to comfort that acknowledges an afterlife may or may not be comforting.

Diet and Lifestyle: Prescriptions and Proscriptions

Kosher directives are interpreted with great diversity; they may be fully observed or not observed at all. For example, a Reform Jew may eat anything except pork, or be a vegetarian or vegan, or interpret law to mean to avoiding gluttony, unethically produced food of any sort, and meat that was cruelly killed. Thus:

- Assess what are acceptable foods for each liberal-minded Jew.

Additional Miscellaneous Nursing Implications

If a Jewish patient cannot communicate his or her preferences, provide care that observes traditional practices (see Chapters 24 and 25 on Conservative and Orthodox Judaism).

Ways and Words to Comfort

Spoken Jewish prayers would typically be considered inappropriate for a non-Jewish nurse to offer. If, however, there is no Jew to pray on behalf of the patient, the patient may appreciate a YouTube rendition of a Jewish prayer for healing (e.g., www.youtube.com/watch?v=NxXQzfTHnV4) or a printout of such prayers (e.g., Barlev, n.d.; Klein, n.d.) or a Jewish prayer offered by a non-Jewish chaplain.

- Prayers and blessings for daily life are available on the Reform Judaism website (https://reformjudaism.org/practice/prayers-blessings). They provide insight about how a Jew prays when ill or distressed.
- A nurse's prayer in any language, however, that asks for healing or comfort will be appreciated by a Jewish patient who requests it. Addressing the divine "God" or "Lord" would be acceptable.
- If present for a prayer, do not kneel or make the sign of the cross (or portray your religious behavior, as it may be interpreted as disrespectful); instead, bow the head while standing. Saying "amen" (pronounced ah MAYN) after a prayer is respectful—and in Jewish tradition, it gives you credit for saying the prayer.
- Read an appropriate Psalm (collection of poetic prayers in the Hebrew scriptures [known by non-Jews as the Old Testament of the Bible]). For example, read Psalms 16:8–9, 11, or 91 or the first two verses of Psalms 40, 46, or 61, which all describe finding safety and strength in God; Psalm 139:7–8 and the famous Psalm 23 describe God being present in difficult times. An online search for comforting Psalms will produce more reads.
- Show respect for Sabbath and Jewish holidays when possible.

Bibliography

American-Israeli Cooperative Enterprise. (n.d.). *Jewish virtual library.* Retrieved from http://www.jewishvirtuallibrary.org

Barlev, P. (Ed.). (n.d.). *Prayer and readings for comfort and healing.* Los Angeles: UCLA Department of Spiritual Care. Retrieved from http://huc.edu/ckimages/files/Kalsman/Barlev.PDF

Klein, F. L. (Ed.). (n.d.). *Jewish prayers for healing.* Miami, FL: The Jewish Chaplaincy Program of the Greater Miami Jewish Federation of Chaplains. Retrieved from http://jewishmiami.org/about/departments/chaplaincy/Desktop/BrochureDraft8.pdf

My Jewish Learning. (n.d.). *Beliefs & practices.* Retrieved from https://www.myjewishlearning.com/category/study/beliefs-practices/

Union for Reform Judaism. (n.d.). *What is reform Judaism?* Retrieved from https://reformjudaism.org/what-reform-judaism

27

Nation of Islam

Other Names and Similar Religious Traditions

Black Muslims are members of the Nation of Islam (NoI). An off-shoot of NoI, developed by the son of its founder who further aligned it with orthodox (or universal) Islam, is the **American Society of Muslims**.

Social and Historical Background

Islam is the god of persons of African descent, according to the NoI. The Savior (who lived for a time on earth as God/Allah) who understood and taught this and other NoI beliefs was Master Wallace (Fard) Muhammad, who lived from 1877 to an unknown time. From 1931 to 1934 he taught Elijah (Poole) Muhammad who became the first leader, or the Messenger, of NoI. Since 1975, Louis Farrakhan has led the NoI.

Beliefs are similar to Sunni Islamic beliefs, with variation. Although the NoI observe the "five pillars of Islam" (see Chapter 23), mainstream Islam does not accept that Fard or Elijah Muhammad were the Messianic Prophet and Messenger, respectively, nor do they accept the Black supremacist stance of NoIs. Furthermore, it is not unusual for NoI ministers to quote Christian scripture, suggesting NoI is a syncretic blending of Islam and Christianity.

Although this stance has softened in more recent years, NoI members believe that Black peoples are the original and superior race. While Blacks have been thought to represent good—indeed, Allah—Whites represent evil. It is believed that it is a sin to integrate with the rebel nation (United States) that enslaved Black peoples; given this,

NoI members advocate and use nonviolent means to promote Black well-being and justice.

Worship and Devotional Practices

Like Muslims, Black Muslims pray five times per day, pay alms for the poor, travel to Mecca for the hajj (if possible during one's lifetime), and observe the fast of Ramadan (but do so during December). Although they often quote the Bible as well as the Quran, neither are believed to be holy scripture. They find religious instruction from the writings and recordings of NoI leaders Elijah Muhammad and Louis Farrakhan as well as their local clergy. The denomination's journal and books are available for purchase at www.noi.org/final-call-news. Savior's Day (January 26), the birth of the Master of NoI, is celebrated with a large livestreamed convention where NoI leaders speak.

- If traveling for the hajj, provide healthcare that informs and protects the patient from potential health-related issues (see Chapter 23).
- Support patients unable to independently complete the prayers five times daily (see Chapter 23).

Illness and Healing: Beliefs and Practices

The body is the metaphorical "temple of God." The founder of NoI identified seven "mind dimensions" of persons: the physical, emotional, mental, spiritual, soul, self, and will. Thus, one's spirituality is a part of one's whole being, and whole person health is valued. The admonitions for healthful living eschewed by Elijah Muhammad are offered in his books titled *How to Eat to Live* (available for purchase at the NoI publisher Final Call, store.finalcall.com/collections/how-to-eat-to-live).

The slavery of Blacks in the United States and their ensuing marginalization continues to affect their health today. NoI leaders recognize that the epidemics of obesity, diabetes, heart disease, and other chronic illnesses that plague impoverished or poorly informed Blacks contribute to their poor health. Food deserts, chemically toxic environments, disparities in healthcare access, and so forth explain disproportionate rates of chronic illness among Blacks.

Beginning of Life: Beliefs and Practices

Strong proscriptions exist against premarital sex and interracial marriage. Indeed, sex with a non-Black (especially a White person) is forbidden. Large families are encouraged; birth control is thought to prevent women from performing their duty to procreate. Men are the protectors of women and may chaperone them.

End of Life: Beliefs and Practices

There will be a "mental resurrection" for the righteous who die. Blacks will be resurrected first. End-of-life beliefs of NoI are not readily available; therefore, when appropriate, inquire of NoI members regarding how they want end-of-life care to be.

Diet and Lifestyle: Prescriptions and Proscriptions

How to Eat to Live (written by the founder of NoI) influences the diet and lifestyle of NoI members. Although some NoI members may not yet incorporate his health teachings, others aspire to do so. Salient points offered in these books include:

- Healthful living involves eating one meal per day (between 4 and 6 p.m.); for those who are unable or sick, two meals per day should suffice.
- Pork, smoking, alcohol, and abusive substances are never to be consumed.
- Although a plant-based diet is the ideal, if meat is to be eaten, consider scavengers, fowl, and red meats more deleterious than white meats, dairy products, and fish (less than 10 pounds heavy).
- Eat lots of fresh fruit and vegetables. Fruits are defined as any edible plant with seeds (e.g., squash, tomatoes). Vegetables must be cooked; that is, they must be steamed, not boiled. (Sweet potatoes are thought to produce gas, and they are avoided.)
- Nuts, legumes, and grains are permitted, but they must be cooked. Grains must be finely ground, and when baked, the bread must rise and be baked twice and then allowed to sit for 3 days. For example, 100% whole grain bread can be eaten if toasted.
- Food should not be cooked in aluminum (or using aluminum foil); stainless steel is recommended.

The understanding and adherence to these dietary recommendations will vary. Even the Messenger Elijah Muhammad admitted he ate meat.

Additional Miscellaneous Nursing Implications

- Modesty is important to women, who should be respected; women cover their heads with "headpieces" (like nuns' habits or

Muslim hijabs); they likewise will wear clothing that covers their arms and legs. Thus, assure modesty and privacy.

■ Homosexuality is believed to be against God's will. NoI lesbian, gay, bisexual, transgender, and queer (LGBTQ) members likely experience considerable inner tension about how to make sense of their sexuality within their beliefs.

Ways and Words to Comfort

■ A classic greeting is "Peace" or "Peace be upon you" (said in Arabic); however, using the English version would also show respect.

Bibliography

Allah, R. (2015). *How to eat to live series, part 1* (the vegetarian diet). Retrieved from https://www.youtube.com/watch?v=TiIqIyv_CGw

Kenneth, D. (2017, Sept. 29). The Nation of Islam on sexual relationships. *Synonym*. Retrieved from https://classroom.synonym.com/the-nation-of-islam-on-sexual-relationships-12086789.html

Muhammad, A. (2006). *Interview with Nation of Islam Minister of Health, Dr. Abdul Alim Muhammad.* December 10. Retrieved from http://www.finalcall.com/artman/publish/Health_amp_Fitness_11/Interview_with_Nation_of_Islam_Minister_of_Health__3096.shtml

Nation of Islam. (n.d.). *Honorable Elijah Muhammad.* Retrieved from https://www.noi.org/hon-elijah-muhammad

Ohm, R. (2003). The African American experience in the Islamic faith. *Public Health Nursing, 20*(6), 478–486. doi:10.1046/j.1525-1446.2003.20608.x

28

"Nones"

Other Names and Similar Religious Traditions

The term *Nones* describes those who self-identify as nonreligious or unaffiliated with a faith tradition; it can include **atheists** (who lack belief in a god[s]), **agnostics** (who are uncertain whether there is a god or accept that such mysteries are not understandable), **freethinkers**, **ethical culturists**, **rationalists**, **skeptics**, and **secular humanists** (who reject religion and superstition in favor of a rational, ethical, scientific philosophical approach to life). They are dubbed "Nones" because they would respond to a religious affiliation question with responses such as "I don't know" or "No religion."

Social and Historical Background

When 35,000 people from across the 50 states of the United States were surveyed, 23% indicated they were "Nones" (Pew Research Center, n.d.). Of these, 16% were "nothing in particular," while 7% identified as atheist or agnostic. These findings represent a steady increase in "Nones" in the United States over the past few decades. "Nones" are more prevalent among those younger than 50 years of age, Whites, those who are not first- or second-generation immigrants, and those who lean Democrat. It may not be surprising that roughly 80% accepted abortion and same-sex marriages and endorsed strong environmental regulation.

Given that most "Nones" in this survey were not atheist or agnostic, these respondents still had some religious inclinations. That is, 60% believed "in God," 33% agreed religion was important in their lives, 38% reported they prayed, and 36% indicated they meditated at least monthly. It is possible that some "Nones" are disenfranchised by institutionalized religion or have unresolved spiritual or religious struggle.

Worship and Devotional Practices

Atheists, agnostics, and secular humanists do form organizations and hold conventions or monthly meetings to discuss their worldviews. Whereas they do not pray to a god, they may practice some forms of meditation and find peacefulness when in nature. Reading philosophy and science as well as discussing such can provide intellectual nurture. Online forums and journals exist for these groups (e.g., *The Freethinker*, *Secular Nation*, and *American Atheist Magazine*).

Illness and Healing: Beliefs and Practices

Atheists and those with similar worldviews do not subscribe to a holistic definition of well-being that includes a spiritual dimension; for other "Nones" who accept a spiritual reality, this will likely be held. Likewise, atheists, agnostics, and secular humanists will reject any supernatural explanations for disease, favoring scientific ones. Likewise, "treatments" without scientific support are unlikely to be followed (e.g., homeopathic remedies, energy channeling, new-age crystals).

- Planning "spiritual care" for an atheist would be inappropriate if it were linked with religiosity. Supporting meaning-making, of course, would be appropriate.

Beginning of Life: Beliefs and Practices

There are no unique beliefs or practices.

End of Life: Beliefs and Practices

For atheists, there is no spiritual reality; therefore, there is no afterlife, angels, ghosts, immortal souls, and so forth. Facing one's death can prompt reflection on what purpose and meaning are experienced in life. Thus:

- Support the exploration of finding meaning. Encourage remembrance of good deeds done, family, and other legacies (e.g., "What are you famous for?" or "When you think about the story of your life, what stands out?").
- It is offensive to an atheist if anyone (e.g., patient's family or friends, nurses) tries to invoke a deathbed conversion. Instead, support the patient to listen to the self speaking by listening deeply and providing therapeutic responses.

Diet and Lifestyle: Prescriptions and Proscriptions

Evidence-informed practices that promote health are appropriate.

Additional Miscellaneous Nursing Implications

- Friends and family may be especially important for "Nones," given they do not have clergy or fellow believers from which to find support.
- Remove religious symbols from a patient's hospital room, if necessary and appropriate.

Ways and Words to Comfort

- Atheists, agnostics, and secular humanists often experience discrimination in cultures where beliefs in a god(s) and religiosity are prevalent. Thus, nonjudgmental and nonevangelistic responses to spiritual struggles will show respect.
- Offering to pray with or for an atheist would be insulting. Indications of personal caring, however, can still be shown (e.g., presence, caring touch, knowing look, or stating "You'll be in my heart and thoughts . . .").
- When comforting an atheist, refrain from religious language; this would be rude.
- If a dying atheist's visitor is trying to proselytize the patient, it may cause distress for both the patient and visitor. Nurses can ascertain whom the patient wants to see and support those nearest to the patient. A patient distressed by someone proselytizing may need to debrief with a therapeutic nurse. Likewise, a nurse may provide emotional support to the disappointed proselytizer by listening empathically so insight can be gained.

Whereas these nursing implications are primarily for the atheist, discretion is needed to determine how to relate to the "Nones" who yet believe in a god(s), prayer, and so forth. Listen to the language used, assess what spiritual needs and resources exist, and then determine appropriate, sensitive responses.

Bibliography

American Atheists. (n.d.). *What is atheism?* Retrieved from https://www.atheists.org/activism/resources/about-atheism

Edwords, F. (2008). *What is Humanism?* American Humanist Association. Retrieved from https://americanhumanist.org/what-is-humanism/edwords-what-is-humanism

Exline, J. J., Park, C. L., Smyth, J. M., & Carey, M. P. (2011). Anger toward God: Social-cognitive predictors, prevalence, and links with adjustment to bereavement and cancer. *Journal of Personal & Social Psychology,* *100*(1), 129–148. doi:10.1037/a0021716

Pew Research Center. (n.d.). *Religious landscape study.* Retrieved from http://www.pewforum.org/religious-landscape-study

Silverman, D. (2012). *Atheists.* In E. J. Taylor (Ed.), *Religion: A clinical guide for nurses* (pp. 117–122). New York, NY: Springer Publishing.

29

North American Indigenous Religions

Whereas most indigenous (native or aboriginal) peoples do not institutionalize their religiosity, their cultures inevitably are interwoven with religiosity. This chapter attempts to provide a cursory look at religiosity among the indigenous of North America: the Native Americans and Alaskans and the First Nations people. The chapter offers general and broad guidelines that are not specific to any indigenous group. Many of the generalizations about North American indigenous people may be applicable to the Maori and Australian aboriginal peoples who were likewise colonized and dominated by Europeans. Thus:

- Consult trusted resources regarding the specific tribal nation of a patient to provide religio-culturally sensitive care.
- Assess each Native American patient for spiritual/religious beliefs and practices pertinent to health.

Other Names and Similar Religious Traditions

The **Native American Church**, or **Peyote Church**, is an umbrella organization for a network of local groups holding spiritual meetings; officially, it is the **Oklevueha Lakota Sioux Native American Church**. Other indigenous North American religious movements include the **Indian Shaker** (in the Pacific Northwest), the **Longhouse Tradition** (northeast), and the **Ghost Dance** (central).

Social and Historical Background

In North America, there are over 600 indigenous tribes. Given this, there is great diversity of religiosity. Whereas some maintain ancient rituals, others adopt rituals that reflect events of modern times. Likewise, there is variation in how indigenous peoples relate to Christianity, the religion of the colonizers. Whereas some become Christian, others completely oppose Christianity, and others blend Christianity with indigenous beliefs and practices in various ways. Regardless, religiosity offers indigenous peoples a means for continuing traditions and identity as well as a means for addressing the racism and poverty resulting from colonialism and imperialism.

Although there are substantial variations, some commonalities exist. First, there is an integration of sacred and secular (e.g., there is not a word for "religion" in some indigenous languages; all of life is considered suffused with spirituality, albeit in different amounts). Second, because there is an animating spiritual power in all of nature, the natural environment and its features (e.g., mountains, springs, animals) are to be respected and appreciated—for some, treated as relatives; harmony with them nurtures one's spirit and ensures human survival. Third, religiosity is typically expressed communally; harmonious relations between living persons and those in a spirit world (unborn or passed on) are sought. Religious rituals are often performed in a group; group meetings (e.g., tribal councils) typically begin with prayer. Fourth, religio-cultural knowledge, whether the story of creation and the cosmos, purification rituals, or other beliefs and practices, is typically shared via an oral tradition in stories, songs, art, and dance. Fifth, tribal elders (and occasionally, prophets) are involved in the community at the request of the family. Sixth, individual, tribal, or intertribal ceremonies are central to indigenous religiosity; they often provide meaning for major life events such as birth, naming, adoption, puberty, marriage, and death.

Worship and Devotional Practices

For some indigenous peoples, there is sacredness in all the natural world and meaningful objects or places within it may be revered. Some indigenous peoples also worship various supernatural beings. These include but are not limited to Great Spirit (or Great Mystery) as the creator god, Mother Earth, Father Sky, and a variety of other supernatural beings. For some indigenous peoples, these other supernatural beings are often described as good or well intentioned, though dangerous if treated carelessly or with disrespect. Although indigenous religions are oral traditions, sacred texts do exist; however, they would not be shared across tribes or nations. Thus:

- When appropriate, inquire if there are tribal-specific supernatural beings that may affect one's health.
- A patient may find wisdom in the collection of Native American myths archived by Hare (2010), available at www.sacred-texts .com/nam/index.htm. Books with Native American legends, prayers, songs, and stories of healing are available (e.g., *Meditations With the Cherokee* [Garrett, 2001]; *American Indian Prayers and Poetry* [Sharpe, 2014]).

Ceremonies generally occur when there is a perceived need (e.g., illness, need to interpret a dream, need to cleanse negative energy) or to mark a significant life event or event in the natural world (e.g., solstice, harvest). Because the sacred is imbued in all of life, however, activities of daily living (e.g., fishing, arising and closing of the day, hunting, cooking) or being in ceremonial spaces (e.g., communal, ceremonial gatherings/dances/feasts, burial grounds) may also contain spiritual meaning. Ceremonies often are held outdoors at a location holding spiritual significance, but they may also be held indoors in a longhouse or tipi. Ritual practices of a ceremony may include, but are not limited to, the following: praying; smudging, singing, or chanting; drumming; dancing; passing a ceremonial object around the group convened; listening to elders' stories and wisdom; burning, smoking, or consuming sacred medicine; and feasting at the conclusion. To prepare for a ceremony, an individual may observe a fast from food or intercourse or detoxify in a sweat lodge. Thus:

- Smudging involves burning a sacred medicine such as sage, cedar, sweetgrass, or lavender and fanning it onto one's body or an object so as to purify it from negative energy. If a hospitalized indigenous patient wants smudging, find an outdoor or negatively ventilated closed space for it. If the patient has a respiratory condition that might contradict the inhalation of smoke, offer a mask. The ceremonial requisites, however, must meet the holy person's specifications.
- Although there are variations in how they are implemented, sweat lodge ceremonies involve heating stones until they are extremely hot, bringing them into a darkened and specially prepared place, and pouring water or fragrant teas over the hot rocks so as to create steam. During this ceremony, attendees offer rounds of intense prayer. The outcome for participants may not only be a cleansing of mind, body, and spirit, but also a sense of community with fellow participants. There may be other purposes for this

experience that are individual to each person, situation, and tribe. As necessary, advise patients considering fasting or a sweat lodge ceremony regarding helpfulness of preceding fasting with a low glycemic diet or the need to retain electrolyte equilibrium if sweating profusely (e.g., push fluids, have salty food). Some may need to be advised not to undergo the sweat ceremony at all (e.g., patients who are pregnant or live with epilepsy, hypertension, or heart disease). Only persons knowledgeable about this ceremony should advise regarding safe participation. Some precautions include that a sweat lodge participant ought to be confident of the ability of the holy man who "pours the waters" on the hot rocks to create the steam and ought to be able to leave the structure if feeling unsafe.

- Some (i.e., not all) indigenous religious ceremonies involve smoking, drinking, or eating tobacco or hallucinogenic plants (e.g., cannabis, ayahuasca, peyote). Tobacco, considered a highly sacred plant, is briefly smoked during some ceremonies for spiritual reasons. Ceremonial tobacco use typically is, and should be, guided by the tribal holy person. Not all tribal nations, however, use these botanicals. The hallucinogens are consumed to create an awareness of oneness with others and to be inspired to a better way of life; sometimes they provide helpful visions. Sometimes these plants are consumed for specific health reasons, but often they are consumed for spiritual reasons just as the Eucharist is in Christian traditions. They are legal in the United States if consumed only within the context of a Native American Church.

- Understand that dreams may provide the dreamer with psycho-spiritual insight. If a patient appears to want to discuss a dream, listen deeply and respectfully, without interpretation. Refer the patient to their holy person for guidance. If a dream is shared with the nurse, understand this is an indication of the person placing great trust in the nurse.

Illness and Healing: Beliefs and Practices

To be well, indigenous patients will seek harmony and balance; they and their communities will strive to fulfill any religio-cultural obligations. Causes of disease or disability include "spirit loss" (departure of one's guardian spirit); sorcery; negative spiritual energy (e.g., from anger, grief); and other natural factors. Indigenous peoples may consult shamans or medicine people to obtain healing. The cause of the illness, as interpreted by the shaman, will determine the treatment. Thus:

- Healing practices with implications for Western healthcare include the use of various herbs. Inquire as to what herbs or plants are being used concurrent to pharmacological agents, to determine if there are any adverse interactive effects. A respectful relationship is requisite to discussing patient preferences and practices.

- Whereas some may believe pain is to be endured and refuse pain medication, others will accept it. Assess and plan care accordingly.
- Some may not want pictures taken of themselves (e.g., hard copies of ultrasound findings). Likewise, when a body part is removed, it must be properly disposed of after a blessing. Ask the patient if there is a preferred ceremonial way for disposing of the body part.
- Helpful questions to ask include, "Are there any traditional healing practices that I need to be aware of to care for you?" and, "Would you like a medicine man/woman called?"

Beginning of Life: Beliefs and Practices

Historical and social factors may influence a Native American seeking gynecological care. Native American women living on reservations experience not only a high rate of sexual assault and domestic violence against them but also a system that fails to bring justice. Also, Native Americans may also be affected by the memory of 3,400 pure-blooded women who were sterilized against their will by the Indian Health Service in the early 1970s.

For some pregnant Native Americans, it may be customary to observe a "strong" diet; likewise, traditional medicines and herbs may be taken during pregnancy and during the delivery. Rituals may be observed after the delivery. Thus:

- Assess what herbs and medicines are being taken to determine if any are known to have an interactive effect with Western medications that will be prescribed.
- Inquire as to what religio-cultural practices the family desires after the delivery. Negotiate if and how these can be observed (e.g., "Does the umbilical cord need to be preserved?")

End of Life: Beliefs and Practices

End-of-life beliefs and practices vary substantially between tribal nations. Given the sensitivity needed for discussing (or not discussing) this topic with a patient, it is essential that a nurse consult a knowledgeable, cultural resource person who can advise how to provide care. Often, indigenous people view death as part of the cycle of life, a transition to another life where they will be united with their ancestors. Before death, however, it may be believed that discussing an eventual death may hasten it. Some believe that to successfully transition to the next world, the whole body must be present. Thus:

- For some, it is safest to talk about death in the third person (e.g., "When persons have this happen to them, they often do not live more than a year" or "How would someone like you want to face the future?").
- Discussing an advance directive could harm not only the nurse's relationship to the patient but also the relationship between the healthcare organization and the patient's tribal community. Discuss advance directives or other aspects of end-of-life care per the advice of the local cultural expert. If appropriate, the discussion could be prefaced with a normalizing statement. For example, "We are required to ask all patients some questions about their preferences; is this something you would like to talk about? Or would you prefer I ask your family?" Remember that some may not want this to be discussed at all and would consider this a hindrance toward their healing.

At the time of death, some may believe they should not be present, and some may believe it is important to be at the bedside. Grief may not be expressed in the presence of the dying. Also, the dying patient may want to have a clear mind at the time of death, so he or she may refuse analgesics; some, however, will want to receive effective pain management. Thus:

- Assess beliefs and preferences regarding pain management at the end of life.
- Do not construe lack of expressed sadness as a failure to grieve. Opportunities to discuss emotions when away from the bedside will likely be appreciated.

After a death, there may be specific rituals or practices. For example, some may want a window open and the patient's name never spoken so that the spirit can more easily transition. Thus:

- Assess what rituals and practices the patient's family will observe that require support from the clinicians. Respectfully provide that support.
- Bereavement beliefs of traditional and contemporary tribal members will vary significantly

Diet and Lifestyle: Prescriptions and Proscriptions

Diet and lifestyle will vary within and between the many indigenous tribes. Many indigenous peoples live in economically and ecologically impoverished conditions. Healthful food and water sources may be scant. Alcoholism rates are often higher for indigenous peoples, as are diabetes and heart disease. Diet will therefore reflect what they are able to obtain as well as cultural traditions. There may be customs about what foods are to be eaten during certain times of the day, season, or transitions in life (e.g., pregnancy, illness). Thus:

- Assess if the patient is observing any special diet.
- When providing health education, first determine what foods and pertinent resources are available as well as what pertinent beliefs may exist.

Additional Miscellaneous Nursing Implications

- The culturally sensitive nurse will utilize trusted resources or resource persons of the specific tribal nation of their patient before caring for the Native American.
- The term *family* can include persons not defined by the "White culture" as family. Therefore, accept the patient's definition of who is included as a family member.
- Major healthcare decisions may be made by the family or community. Be receptive to tribal elders' input.
- Communication is not always with words. For many tribal nations, silence is an important way of communicating. Be sensitive to the use of silence; listen and do not interrupt, as this is considered by many tribal nations as highly offensive. Silence to ponder conveys respect for the speaker. Silence before one's response indicates that the words are carefully considered before speaking.
- Provide a space for spiritual items to be placed at the bedside.

Ways and Words to Comfort

- For many different tribes and traditions, the drum is a powerful and resonant symbol of Indian identity and spirituality. For some tribal nations, the drum sings the heartbeat of mother earth. It is considered the unified connection of all beings and the cosmos. Facilitating a patient to listen to a recording of drumming may be comforting. Recordings are available on compact disks (www .native-languages.org/drums.htm) and free on iTunes, YouTube, and Spotify.
- If the patient's beliefs are substantially Christian, a prayer or reading in the appendix may be comforting.
- If the patient's religion is substantially Christian and prayer is requested, the nurse can offer a prayer or reading in the appendix.
- Ask if there is a spiritual advisor the patient would like to have called.

Bibliography

Aboriginal Spirituality. (n.d.). *The faith project*. Retrieved from http://the faithproject.nfb.ca/wp-content/uploads/2015/03/TFP_Aboriginal_Dec 2014.pdf

Dees, S. E. (2018). Native American religions. *Oxford Religious Encyclopedias*. doi:10.1093/acrefore/9780199340378.013.404.

Garrett, J. T. (2001). *Meditations with the Cherokee: Prayers, songs, and stories of healing and harmony*. Rochester, NY: Bear & Co.

Hare, J. B. (2010). *Native American religions. Internet sacred text archive*. Retrieved from http://sacred-texts.com/nam/index.htm

Isaacson, M. J. (2018). Addressing palliative and end-of-life care needs with Native American elders. *International Journal of Palliative Nursing, 24*(4), 160–168. doi:10.12968/ijpn.2018.24.4.160

Oklevuaha Native American Church. (n.d.). *Spirituality*. Retrieved from https://nativeamericanchurches.org/spirituality

President and Fellows of Harvard College, Eck, D. (n.d.). *Native American traditions*. The Pluralism Project/Harvard University. Retrieved from http://pluralism.org/religions/native-american-traditions

Sharpe, J. E. (2014). *American Indian prayers and poetry*. Cherokee, NC: Cherokee Publications.

Smith, D. G., Parrott, Z., & Felice, M. (2018). *Religion and spirituality of indigenous peoples in Canada*. The Canadian Encyclopedia. Retrieved from https://www.thecanadianencyclopedia.ca/en/article/religion-of-aboriginal-people

Tanenbaum Center for Interreligious Understanding. (2009). *The medical manual for religio-cultural competence* (pp. 164–176). New York, NY: Author.

30

Sikhism

Other Names and Similar Religious Traditions

Because most Sikhs are of South Asian descent and Sikh men often wear turbans and have long beards, Westerners may confuse them with Muslims or adherents of other South Asian religions.

Social and Historical Background

Sikhism originated around 1500 in northern (Punjab) India, when a guru had a mystical experience that revealed spiritual insights that differed from those of the prevailing religions of the region (i.e., Islam and Hinduism). Over the next 200 years, a series of succeeding gurus provided leadership, wrote holy literature, and further developed beliefs and practices. Sikhs (or those who are disciples of God) worship a monotheistic God, *Waheguru/Vahiguru* or *Akal Purukh*, a timeless being who created and sustains the universe and is also attentive to each person—a divine parent. The core values of Sikhism include work (making an honest living), charity (serving the community), and worship (remembering God). The purpose of life is to live virtuously so as to prepare the soul for union with God. Social interactions reflect Sikhs' espousal that all are equal to God, regardless of their gender, race, religion, and so forth.

Worship and Devotional Practices

The gurdwara is the temple where Sikhs gather to worship, to socialize, and to organize themselves to serve the community. For instance, gurdwaras provide the space where members can collectively prepare and share food for themselves and anybody who needs help; free vegetarian Indian meals are offered all day every day! Gurdwaras are open every day, yet many may frequent them only on Sundays. A religious service will involve hymn singing, a homily, recitations of prayers, and distribution of "sanctified food." The spiritual leader of a gurdwara is the granthi, a Sikh scholar knowledgeable about rituals and scripture. Thus:

- Bedbound Sikhs will likely greatly miss their gurdwara's community experience. Local Sikhs, however, will likely visit often given it is an encouraged spiritual act.
- If an ethical decision is faced, engage the granthi if the patient desires.

The 10th guru decreed that the compiled religious writings of these founding gurus would be the succeeding and everlasting guru. Thus, these hymns, prayers, and other holy literature constitute the nearly 1,500-page Guru Granth Sahib (or Adi Granth), Sikh's holy scriptures. The *Rehat Maryada*, composed by a committee, is not a sacred text but provides believers with a code of conduct and describes how various life events and rituals should be observed. Many Sikh family homes will have a room for the Guru Granth Sahib. Sikhs communicate with God/Waheguru through prayer (usually recited from the scripture) individually and collectively as well as by meditating on the divine name. Specific prayers are recited at different times of the day (i.e., predawn, dusk, and just before bedtime). Thus:

- The posture of prayer is one of sitting, although the final prayers are said while standing. Prayers are preceded by cleansing: hands are washed (with running water, if possible); mouth is rinsed; footwear removed; and head covered. If clothing is soiled, it should be replaced. Inquire of patients as to how assistance may be provided. Determine also at what time they will pray so that interruptions can be avoided.
- Given prayers are recited, baptized Sikhs will always have with them a small book of prayers. This sacred book needs to be respected by maintaining its cleanliness; if the patient permits the nurse to handle it, the nurse must wash hands or don gloves first.
- For those who do not have their own prayer book, the scriptural instruction for the day selected at the holiest *gurdwala* (the Golden Temple in Amritsar, India) can be found online at SikhNet's Daily Hukamnama (www.sikhnet.com/hukam).
- Meditating on the name of God (i.e., *Naam*) is another way Sikhs connect with God and find liberation from suffering and salvation. This can mean literally speaking or chanting the name or short prayer repeatedly or silently reflecting on the qualities

of God. Whatever approach taken, Sikhs typically meditate while sitting cross-legged with hands together. Inquire if a patient would like to schedule uninterrupted time for meditation.

- If a patient wears prayer beads around the wrist or neck or any other religious items (five Ks, see "Diet and Lifestyle"), treat these with utmost respect when bathing. Avoid removing any worn religious items; do so only when absolutely necessary and it is agreed upon by the patient.

Holidays celebrate the founding of the religion and various gurus' birthdays as well as other historical events important to Sikhs.

Illness and Healing: Beliefs and Practices

Sikhs believe that a soul cycles through many births and deaths before becoming a human; furthermore, one's behaviors in the present life determine how they will be rebirthed (reincarnation). The rebirthing allows purification of the soul, and ultimately the soul can unite with God. Thus, many Sikhs will attribute illness and tragedy to karma, or the result of sins in a previous life. When health challenges arise, therefore, Sikhs may become more fervent in their devotions. They will also seek to balance their spiritual and temporal strivings. Sikhs likely also believe that their disease or disability is in a benevolent God's will. This belief, however, does not mean a fatalistic response; Sikhs believe it is important to seek healthcare and take reasonable action to promote life. Thus:

- Although no healing rituals are practiced, supporting patients' devotional practices is important. In addition to wanting prayer and meditation, patients may want to listen to recordings of sacred Sikh hymns. If earphones are needed, obtain ones that do not disturb a head covering.
- Given the import of prayers while sick and the import of cleansing prior to these and for healing, a Sikh patient may be extremely eager to shower every morning prior to daybreak.
- Although suffering is viewed as a test of one's ability to live in "high spirits," Sikhs will accept pain medications and analgesics.

Because many Sikhs are from (or influenced by) the culture of the Punjab region, decision making will occur as is common in a collectivist society. Thus:

- Consult Sikh patients as to who they would like to have involved in decision making (e.g., family members, granthi). Plan discussions about a decision with these persons present.

Mental health concerns are typically stigmatized. Seeking counseling is often considered taboo, as the Sikh is seen to be seeking help from outside the family and Sikh community. Thus:

- When possible, make referrals to Sikh mental health professionals or those who understand the dynamics of living within a tightly knit community.

Beginning of Life: Beliefs and Practices

Although Sikh teachings do admonish baptized members to not be adulterous and to not circumcise, perinatal issues are generally determined individually and influenced by culture, rather than religion. When a child is born, the mother may loathe having the infant removed from her. She may also choose to not take the baby out in public for 40 days. After this period, the baby will be taken to the gurdwala for a naming ceremony. Thus:

- Initial postnatal check-ups may need to be performed in the home.
- Make accommodation if the parents are not willing to provide a name for the baby.
- Assess for religio-cultural determinants influencing perinatal decisions when needed.

If a miscarriage or stillbirth occurs, wrap the fetus in a clean white cloth, and present it to the family for bathing and cremation. Do not cut any hair off the fetus.

End of Life: Beliefs and Practices

The body is thought of as a "shell" for the soul; it is temporary for the present life. Thus, the soul of the dedicated, virtuous Sikh who dies goes to heaven to be united with God. For those who did not live as obedient Sikhs, the cycle of reincarnation will continue. Respect for all at the time of death is provided, given no one knows any soul's future. Thus:

- Euthanasia, assisted suicide, and prolonged artificial life support for a patient in a vegetative state are discouraged. Religio-cultural mores influencing such decisions will vary and need to be assessed when needed.
- Organ transplantation and autopsies are generally acceptable.
- When offering "condolences," focus on what was appreciated in the deceased; while sadness will inevitably be felt, some Sikhs may prefer to focus on the joy of the deceased's soul merging with God. Follow cues so as to be empathic.

When dying is imminent, the patient's family (or Sikh representatives) should be at the bedside to recite scripture and prayers. Sacred hymns from scripture are often sung; if Sikhs are not present or able to sing, recordings of these hymns are available and can be played at the bedside of the dying. After the death, scriptural hymns will also be recited by the Sikhs present. Thus:

- Nurses can welcome those gathered at the bedside and try to provide a private environment where the recitations and music can be offered.
- Obtain from the Sikh family the means for playing hymns the patient would want played in the patient's absence, if needed. Obtain clearance for any electronic devices, per institution policy.

After the death, support Sikh practices. Thus:

- Do not remove any religious items that the patient wore, or return them to the body if they were removed.
- Do not bathe or dress the body; this is a role for family members. If this is to occur at a funeral home, perform otherwise usual postmortem care, and encase the body in clean linens and the shroud. For males, neatly arrange the hair in a knot above the head, and cover with their turban.

Diet and Lifestyle: Prescriptions and Proscriptions

Sikhs who are baptized are expected to maintain several practices. Alcohol, tobacco, and nonmedicinal drugs are strictly forbidden, as are cutting one's hair, eating meat, and committing adultery. A vegetarian diet, which likely will include dairy products (except eggs), is followed. Sikhs who are not yet baptized may or may not observe these practices. For Sikhs who do eat meat, they may observe rules regarding how the meat is prepared (e.g., they will not eat meat slaughtered following kosher or halal procedures). Thus:

- Unless specified otherwise by the Sikh patient, order a vegan or lacto-vegetarian diet. Do not order halal or kosher food. Inform patient/family if there are any dietary restrictions or policies regarding bringing food in, as it is likely food will be brought from home.
- Ensure that medications are free of meat by-products (e.g., porcine gelatin).

A Sikh who chooses to live the disciplined life as described in the code of conduct is baptized.

Baptized Sikhs, or Khalsa, are given a name at the baptism to denote their commitment: Singh (for men); Kaur (for women). The code of conduct also stipulates that Khalsa wear external symbols of their religion. These symbols include hair that is to never be cut (*kesh*); a wooden comb worn in the hair (*kanga*); a miniature sword (kirpan)—typically worn under clothing; an iron wrist ring (*kara*); and an undergarment that covers the pelvis and thighs (*kachh*). A non-Khalsa Sikh may wear these as well. Because these elements all begin with *k*, they are collectively called the five Ks. Although younger and Westernized Sikhs are redefining how to observe their religious code, the five Ks do make obvious indicators of Sikh identity. Thus:

- Because the hair is never to be cut, it grows very long. Men twist it into a knot above their head and cover it with a turban. Women cover their heads with a turban or headscarf. As needed, assist the Khalsa patient to comb and rearrange his or her hair daily. If needing to remove the turban, respectfully asking for permission to touch the turban will decrease potential anxiety the patient may have in this regard. Do not place it next to shoes or on the floor. An alternative head covering such as a surgical cap will be appreciated.

- Never shave or cut any hair (facial or otherwise) without the patient's permission. Clipping hair for surgery is permitted. Discuss the hair removal, however, prior to surgery. Loss of hair can distress Khalsa as it signifies a breach of spiritual commitment and destroys a symbol of honor. This discussion requires much sensitivity and respect.

- The other worn objects (comb, dagger, wrist ring, and undergarment) are to never be removed unless permission is granted. (To indicate how strongly the intent to maintain religious adherence can be, know that some Sikh women delivering a baby who do not want to remove their undergarment may keep it on one leg. Sometimes Khalsa will not attend events where they are expected to remove their kirpan.)

Additional Miscellaneous Nursing Implications

- Cleanliness is a high priority for Sikhs. Be particularly attentive to hygienic needs and keep the body clean. Wash hair (including beards) as necessary. Comb hair at least daily.

- Respect modesty. If possible, provide nurses of the same gender as the Sikh patient. Provide patient gowns that cover the body well. Knock on a patient's door and announce your arrival. Limit unnecessary touching. Keep patient clothed/gowned as much as possible while conducting an assessment.

Ways and Words to Comfort

- A Sikh may desire to listen to recordings of hymn singing. A nurse can arrange with the help of the family to play such hymns for the patient or find some on YouTube.
- Ask the patient if a reading or prayer would be helpful; if it is desired, assess what would be comforting. A reading of a prayer found on the Internet in English (see www.thoughtco.com/sikh-hymns-offering-encouragement-2993129) or possibly a prayer offered in the nurse's own religious tradition may be welcome.

Bibliography

Ahluwalia, M. K., & Mohabir, R. K. (2017). Turning to Waheguru: Religious and cultural coping mechanisms of bereaved Sikhs. *Omega - Journal of Death and Dying, 78*(3), 302–313. doi:10.1177/0030222816688907

Galdas, P. M., Oliffe, J. L., Kang, H. B., & Kelly, M. T. (2012). Punjabi Sikh patients' perceived barriers to engaging in physical exercise following myocardial infarction. *Public Health Nursing, 29*(6), 534–541. doi:10.1111/j.1525-1446.2012.01009.x

Kalra, G., Bhui, K. S., & Bhugra, D. (2012). Sikhism, spirituality and psychiatry. *Asian Journal of Psychiatry, 5*(4), 339–343. doi:10.1016/j.ajp.2012.08.011

Metropolitan Chicago Healthcare Council. (2000). *Guidelines for health care providers interacting with patients of the Sikh religion and their families.* Retrieved from https://www.advocatehealth.com/assets/documents/faith/cgsikh.pdf

Sikhs.org. (2011). *Introduction to Sikhism.* Retrieved from http://www.sikhs.org/summary.htm

Tanenbaum Center for Interreligious Understanding. (2009). *The medical manual for religio-cultural competence: Caring for religiously diverse populations* (pp. 123–136). New York, NY: Author.

31

Traditional Chinese Religions

Other Names and Similar Religious Traditions

Traditional Chinese religions include **Confucianism**, **Taoism** (**Daoism**), and other folk religions. **Buddhism** (see Chapter 4) also deeply influences Chinese and other Asian cultures. Chinese, Koreans, Japanese, Vietnamese, and other East Asians—and non-Asians who are practitioners of traditional Chinese religions—however, typically will not view themselves as religious (i.e., Taoist or Confucian).

Social and Historical Background

Chinese religious beliefs and behaviors will reflect a blend of these religions. Indeed, among Westernized Chinese, these religious orientations may also be blended with acceptance of Buddhism, Christianity, democracy, or science. These traditional Chinese religions are not institutionalized or codified; furthermore, given the busy lifestyle and inability to read traditional Chinese, practitioners often do not possess a deep understanding of these traditions.

The origins of Confucianism are often attributed to Confucius (551–479 BCE); however, his writings were his attempt to collect and transmit existing Chinese values. The pursuit of human perfection (or realizing one's full potential) is the purpose of living. For Confucians, this is sought through individual effort, such as becoming educated and aware (i.e., about poetry, art, and music; how we communicate with others; history; politics; ecology); developing or supporting art; and being a responsible, virtuous, and serious person. These pursuits are internally motivated, not externally by society or a divinity. Also, integral to Confucianism is the veneration of ancestors and harmonious relationships with family and others in society. Indeed, five types of relationship are recognized, and there is a hierarchy of value for them. In order of importance, these relationships are between parents and children, husband and wife, sibling and sibling or friend and friend, teacher and student, and ruler and subject. Thus, parents, husbands, teachers, and rulers are considered more important than their counterparts, and parents are to be more honored than teachers and rulers. By seeking human perfection in these ways, one not only develops personally but also supports family, society, and all humankind. Likewise, by helping family, society, and humankind, the individual is perfected.

The sacred texts giving rise to Taoism were likely written no earlier than the 2nd or 3rd century (CE); however, they are documentations of the philosophy generated several centuries prior. Taoism offers "a Way" (tao) for achieving holistic well-being. Fundamentally, this wholeness involves a balance of yin and yang. While yin represents the feminine, receptivity, stillness, regression, and so forth, yang represents the masculine, activity, movement, and aggression. People are to seek both yin and yang and keep them in balance—in themselves, in their relations with others, and with nature. Other Taoist themes include naturalness (illustrated in feng shui, which advises how to design inhabited space that is harmonious with nature); intuition (in addition to rationality); and self-cultivation by avoiding the "rat race," being spontaneous, simple, and unsophisticated.

Interspersed with these religious philosophies in China are diverse folk religions. These religions typically vary by geographic area. They often are animistic (believing spiritual beings exist within natural objects like animals) or shamanistic (having religious persons who can perform divinations and offer counsel or healing) and involve worship of local deities or veneration of the spirits of ancestors.

To summarize, these traditional Chinese religions provide nondogmatic guidance for how to live harmoniously and well—physically, emotionally, and spiritually. More important than having the right beliefs is living the right way. Aspects of Confucianism, Taoism, and folk traditions are commonly melded in the lived experience of practitioners.

Worship and Devotional Practices

Because of the strong value for respecting one's elders, practitioners typically venerate their ancestors. They may do so by bowing (with incense in hand) and providing gifts (typically, food) to an altar at home every day. They will also keep their ancestors' gravesites tidy.

They may also visit a community temple, especially on anniversaries and holy days. Practitioners may pray to deities to request advice or protection. Priests/priestesses at a temple may be consulted; some may conduct divinations so as offer counsel from the gods or spirits.

In Western cultures where there are fewer temples, devotional practices are more likely to include reading of Taoist and Confucian sacred texts, of which there are several. Likewise, devotional practices are more likely to focus on holistic methods for achieving health.

Illness and Healing: Beliefs and Practices

Per traditional Chinese thinking, the causes of illness and misfortune are several. They include retribution or being cursed by others who are angry with the patient, living where natural and built environment are imbalanced (poor feng shui), bad luck, an imbalance (within the body or between a person and others or nature), a spiritual or cosmic disharmony, and ghosts or demons. Thus, to seek advice and healing, one may seek out a priest/priestess or feng shui expert, consult astrology or numerology, determine if he or she has failed to perform certain rituals, or obtain an analysis of factors contributing to an imbalance. Thus:

- Those strongly ascribing to these traditional beliefs (e.g., first-generation immigrants) may delay entering Western healthcare until their illness is acute or death is imminent. If there is an interpretation of illness that they are being punished or that they have failed to live according to religious values, there may be significant spiritual or emotional distress.
- Assess what traditional Chinese treatments have been implemented. Diet and herbs are often prescribed by traditional healers and may have interactive effects with prescribed Western pharmaceuticals. (Other traditional Chinese therapies include acupressure, acupuncture, moxibustion, and cupping. These are unlikely to interfere with Western therapeutics.)
- To understand what the patient believes will bring healing, assess with questions like, "What do you do to bring harmony and balance for yourself?"

Beginning of Life: Beliefs and Practices

The following beliefs and practices pertaining to the perinatal period reflect traditional Chinese culture, which is influenced by religion. These include:

- Prenatal dietary proscriptions may include pineapple or lamb; prescriptions may include herbs, chicken broth, and other soups.

- During delivery, a mother or mother-in-law may attend the patient, rather than the father of the newborn. The patient may believe she should not scream during labor.

- After a birth, the infant should not be adored, as this is thought to cause malevolent spirits to cause harm to the infant. Some may believe an infant should not be dressed in previously worn clothing; inquire if the hospital clothing is acceptable.

- Postpartum women may take days or weeks to recover, purposefully resting, wearing warm pajamas, limiting showers, eating certain foods, and keeping windows closed, so as to reestablish balance between what is considered hot and cold. Assess beliefs about what allows recovery, and plan care accordingly. For example, teach range of motion exercises if the patient believes she should remain in bed, and bring food she prefers. An attitude of displeasure toward such a patient "playing the sick role" is inappropriate. Note that family members may believe they should not eat in the presence of a woman with lochial discharge.

End of Life: Beliefs and Practices

If one has lived a moral life, there is no reason to fear death—a natural part of life. Although Confucian writings do not describe an afterlife, Taoists believe a supernatural immortality can be achieved by those who have closely followed the Way of Tao up to the time of death. Nevertheless, practitioners typically believe that speaking about death will hasten it and thinking about it will cause inner disharmony. Thus:

- Follow patient and family cues regarding language to use in discussing dying, and with whom to discuss end-of-life decisions. To begin this assessment, use open questions: "What are your thoughts about your (your parents') future?" "Whom would you like to have involved in making decisions about your future?"

A good death is important, as it will not displease the spirits and cause them to create bad luck for the family later. Whereas some may prefer to die at home, many believe dying in an institution allows for better care and does not bring misfortune to the household. Thus:

- Hospice may be undesirable unless there is an inpatient unit.

End-of-life decisions, ultimately, will be guided by what cultivates morality. If moral value can still be achieved, life should be continued even in the face of great suffering. If, however, there is physical suffering that prevents moral self-cultivation, then it is permissible to choose death. Thus:

- Select therapeutics and dosing so that symptom management can allow this moral growth.

Death rituals vary but will likely involve: (a) the dying patient seeing each family member, (b) announcing the death to the community, (c) washing the body with fresh water so that the deceased's spirit can pass on, (d) placing a lit lamp at the feet of the deceased to light their way; and (e) burial. Thus:

- Before death is imminent, assess what death-related practices may require support.

Living the values of the religion includes filial piety, or letting children honor their parents. Therefore, end-of-life decisions made autonomously would be morally wrong. An advance directive may be viewed as superfluous, yet children may also believe they need to honor their parents by advocating for aggressive therapies to increase longevity. Thus:

- Respect the communication structure requested by the patient. If necessary, allow children requesting futile treatment to verbalize what beliefs prompt this, and guide them to consider other ways of expressing filial piety and what is a good death.

Diet and Lifestyle: Prescriptions and Proscriptions

Given that living long is important to Taoists, Taoism offers a wide range of health-promoting recommendations. These include sleep that is regulated by when the sun shines; regular exercise that involves slow, repetitive motion that stretches the body; exercises for specific parts of the body (e.g., wiggling toes, clicking teeth, squinting eyes); massage; fasting and acts of purification; walking and hiking; breathing mountain or sea air; prayer to the gods of health and longevity; preparing and drinking tea to encourage conversation and relaxation; artistic expression; leisure; meditation and deep breathing that allows one to empty the mind or visualize the divine characteristics; moderate consumption of alcohol; and spending time alone for contemplation. The goal of these practices is to balance qi, the vital energy within persons, thereby restoring its necessary circulation. Thus:

- The above strategies can be incorporated in health promotion education for many East Asians. Some can be introduced during acute care (e.g., art therapy, massage, body stretching motions, meditation).

Additional Miscellaneous Nursing Implications

- Because of the core values of respecting elders and family relationships, healthcare decision making will likely involve not just the patient. Children will often make the decisions for their elderly parents. Respect this family dynamic as a reflection of their benevolence and morality, their "filial piety." Elders will likely approve that discussions about a diagnosis or prognosis be held first with their adult children.

- Similarly, physicians and healthcare providers viewed as authorities may not be countered or questioned.

- It is a virtue to keep inner, private thoughts secret. Thus, East Asian patients may be reluctant to express their ideas. If they do express them and they are rejected, the patient will "lose face," a serious threat to the psyche. To avoid losing face, East Asians may be unassertive, appear to agree even when they do not, and avoid saying no. Nurses can obtain more accurate information, therefore, if they create trust by not disagreeing with the patient or embarrassing them for their perspective and by avoiding yes/no questions.

- Direct eye contact is perceived to be disrespectful; do not interpret it otherwise.

- Control of emotions is also valued; do not interpret stoicism for lack of sorrow or suffering.

Ways and Words to Comfort

- Although these traditional Chinese religions do blend, one may be more manifest than the others. Observe if this is true, and create comforting words as appropriate. The following observations are related to when a death is imminent:
  - For those most influenced by Confucianism, affirm the uprightness and moral character of the one whose life is ending, with assurances that the patient has provided a good model for them all to emulate.
  - For the Taoist, downplay the drama. (A famous story exists of a Taoist sage marking the passing of his beloved wife by beating on a kitchen kettle in a celebratory rhythm.)
  - Buddhists relativize the conclusion of any one lifetime by viewing it as one of many—past and future. They tend to regard the chain of lifetimes as generally ascending; they comfort one another with the thought that such a decent person will surely experience an improved karmic condition next time around (see Chapter 4).

Bibliography

Hsu, C.-Y., O'Connor, M., & Lee, S. (2009). Understandings of death and dying for people of Chinese origin. *Death Studies, 33*(2), 153–174. doi:10.1080/07481180802440431

Nadeau, R. L. (2014). *Asian religions: A cultural perspective*. West Sussex, UK: Wiley Blackwell.

Park, K. H. (2010). Chinese religions. In S. Sorajjakool, M. Carr, & J. J. Nam (Eds.), *World religions for healthcare professionals* (pp. 62–76). New York: Routledge.

The Pluralism Project. (n.d.-a). *The Confucian tradition*. Harvard University. Retrieved from http://pluralism.org/religions/confucianism/the-confucian -tradition

The Pluralism Project. (n.d.-b). *The Daoist tradition*. Harvard University. Retrieved from http://pluralism.org/religions/daoism

Queensland Health. (2018). *Chinese ethnicity and background*. Retrieved from https://www.health.qld.gov.au/__data/assets/pdf_file/0027/158661/chinese -preg-prof.pdf

Tanenbaum Center for Interreligious Understanding. (2009). *The medical manual for religio-cultural competence* (pp. 148–163). New York, NY: Author.

Visscher, C. (2006). Eye on religion: Understanding the cultural/religious mélange in treating Chinese patients. *Southern Medical Journal, 99*(6), 683–684.

32

Zoroastrianism

Other Names and Similar Religious Traditions

Zoroastrians (or **Zarathushti**) living in India are called **Parsees** (or **Parsis**).

Social and Historical Background

Founded by the prophet Zoroaster (or Zarathrustra, c. 1500 BCE), this faith tradition was once the religion of the Persian empire. Now, however, because Zoroastrians were persecuted by their conquerors long ago and lived in societies where it could not be promulgated, it has dwindled to no more than 250,000 worldwide. Indeed, while Zoroastrians do not proselytize, they do accept converts. Although most live in either India or Iran, there are pockets of Zoroastrians in North America and other locations. Generally, Parsees are more ortho-dox in their religious practices than Zoroastrians from Iran. Thus:

- Given the spectrum of Zoroastrian practices, it is important to assess how each patient lives out religious beliefs that have implications for healthcare. Some of the nursing implications identified here may be applicable only to the orthodox Zoroastrian.

The framework for Zoroastrian beliefs is that there are two forces that stand against one another. This battle is spiritual and inter-nal, in one's mind. It manifests externally when the person chooses one side or the other. To achieve perfection and become godlike, Zarathrustra encouraged his followers to choose the forces of good. This is done by making choices to think good thoughts, speak good words, and do good deeds.

Worship and Devotional Practices

Zoroastrians are monotheists, believing in one god, Ahura Mazda ("Wise Lord"). Ahura Mazda is a personal god, a friend. Prayers can occur anytime, anywhere, and without rituals, but the orthodox will pray to Ahura Mazda five times per day (for about 5–10 minutes each time). Prayers are memorized and offered during certain circumstances or times; many prayers are learned during one's youth to prepare for the religious initiation. Prayers are usually recited individually in one's home; however, a believer may attend a temple—especially during festivals. Regardless of location, prayers are said facing of any source of light (open flame, candle, lamp, the sun). The flame symbolizes ultimate wisdom and eternal light. Scriptures (*The Avesta*) include Zarathrustra's own teachings (the *Gathas*) as well as subsequent observances and rules developed by various priests (the *Yashts*, *Dinkard*, *Vendidad*). Thus:

- Most pray by reading prayers from a prayer book (*Khordeh Avesta*) or reciting these from memory. If desired, family or friends can be encouraged to leave a copy at the patient's bedside. Although prayers are typically in their language of origin and the patient may not understand them, they can still create a sense of peace and comfort. The nurse can assist to create a prayerful environment (i.e., assess when the patient wants to pray to protect that time from intrusions, offer an electric candle at night or position to face the sun during the day, provide a head cover if requested [white preferred]).

- If the orthodox patient requests it, assist with the tying of his or her *kusti* (a wool thread) around the waist three times to prepare for prayer.

- Old, but free, issues of the religion's FEZANA Journal are available online at fezana.org/journal-page.

Illness and Healing: Beliefs and Practices

Tragedies such as illness and disability happen because this is the way the earth works. Disease does not occur because of an evil cause; rather it is part of the circle of life. Choosing good will bring the rewards of peace and godlikeness (taking on of Ahura Mazda's characteristics). To not choose good leads to inner chaos. Thus:

- Given beliefs emphasizing thinking good thoughts, speaking good words, and doing good deeds (and working hard), it is possible a Zoroastrian will experience guilt from interpreting illness or disability as a consequence for not having done these things. If guilt or shame is observed, encourage contact with a Zoroastrian priest (*mobed*) or spiritual care expert. A list of priests is available at hamcmobeds.org/directory.

- Free will is important to Zoroastrians. Individuals are to make their own healthcare decisions (e.g., they will not necessarily defer to a priest). Decisions are guided by what will bring goodness and peace to the world.
- Although rarely encountered, some will reject blood transfusions and organ donation, as this would be believed to pollute the Zoroastrian gene pool. When an organ or body part is removed, some will want to dispose of it according to their beliefs.

Beginning of Life: Beliefs and Practices

- For very orthodox practitioners, menstruation is believed to create a state of impurity. Because of this, some women will not go to worship publicly during menses. (In ancient times, there was no means for containing the flow of blood, and it was believed that the blood would potentially transmit disease.) Cleanliness during this time is very important.
- No religious dictates regarding abortion or contraception exist; it is a personal decision.

End of Life: Beliefs and Practices

Zoroastrians believe one can become immortal by living the best and most righteous life possible. Although Zoroaster never described an afterlife, some Zoroastrians believe in a heaven and hell. Most believe heaven or hell to not be a place, but rather a state of the soul. Although there are unique rituals for disposing of the dead in India and Iran, Zoroastrians in North America do bury or cremate the deceased, preferably within 24 hours.

In the final moments of life, friends or family may read certain prayers. Likewise, the dying patient should be dressed in their white muslin shirt (*sudreh*) and have their kusti (a wool thread, prayer cord) around the waist three times. A lit candle, lamp, or incense should be at their head. Thus:

- Ensure the sudreh and kusti are worn at death (if the patient so desires) and after postmortem care.
- If hospitalized, an electric candle will suffice.
- If an organ is to be donated (or an autopsy conducted), coordinate with the personnel so that the organ can be harvested (or autopsy commenced) immediately after death.

Diet and Lifestyle: Prescriptions and Proscriptions

Given most Zoroastrians originate from the Iranian or Indian cultures, their foods may reflect these cultures. There is no prescribed diet. Because the killing of animals "in luxury" is prohibited, however, some Zoroastrians are vegetarians. Parsees may avoid beef.

Additional Miscellaneous Nursing Implications

- Cleanliness is of great importance. Thus, remove body fluids and excreta as soon as possible. This practice, if not observed, may create an irritated patient. Bathe with running water or a freshly drawn water.
- For orthodox Parsees, hair and nails are not to be cut during the nighttime—unless there is need during an emergency.
- Wearing a white muslin shirt (sudreh) with a pocket thought to collect and contain all one's good deeds is always worn next to the skin, day and night. This cloth is not to be cut or removed unless necessary (e.g., bathing, surgery, trauma care). This, as well as the prayer cords, must be treated with respect.
- If removing the prayer cord (kusti), unknot it rather than cutting it—unless it is an emergency.
- On Zoroastrian holidays, practitioners (especially Iranians) will visit the sick. Accommodate the influx if possible.

Ways and Words to Comfort

- It is believed that prayers said as physically close as possible to the patient are more helpful. Thus, facilitate this, if necessary.
- The willing nurse can ask if the patient would like to hear a prayer read (if the patient has an English version of the prayer book). Most would appreciate if a non-Zoroastrian read a prayer for them; however, the more orthodox Zoroastrians (generally, Parsees from India) probably will not want it. The prayer that all Zoroastrians learn first is the *Ashem Vohu*. Translated, it reads, "Righteousness is the best good. It is happiness. Happiness to the one who is righteous for the sake of best righteousness," or "The path of Righteousness is best."

Bibliography

California Zoroastrian Center. (n.d.). *About Zoroastrianism*. Retrieved from https://www.czc.org/about-zoroastrian

Dubash, T. (n.d.). *Keeping the flame alive*. Retrieved from http://www.beliefnet.com/faiths/zoroastrianism/keeping-the-flame-alive.aspx

Greene, J. (1992). Death with dignity: Zoroastrianism. *Nursing Times, 88*(7), 44–45.

Metropolitan Chicago Healthcare Council. (2002). *Guidelines for health care providers interacting with patients of the Zoroastrian/Zarathushti religion and their families*. Retrieved from https://www.advocatehealth.com/assets/documents/faith/cgzoroastrian.pdf

Appendix
Jewish and Christian Prayers
and Readings for the Sick

Christian Prayers

■ Lord's Prayer (in the King James Version, which is acceptable to all Protestant traditions):

Our Father, which art in heaven, Hallowed be thy name. Thy kingdom come. Thy will be done in earth, as it is in heaven. Give us this day our daily bread. And forgive us our debts, as we forgive our debtors. And lead us not into temptation, but deliver us from evil. For thine is the kingdom, and the power, and the glory, for ever. Amen (Matthew 6:9–13).

■ Prayer (by Thomas Merton, a Roman Catholic monk and mystic, in *Thoughts in Solitude*, 1999):

My Lord God, I have no idea where I am going.
I do not see the road ahead of me.
I cannot know for certain where it will end. Nor do I really know myself.
And the fact that I think I am following your will does not mean that I am actually doing so.
But I believe that the desire to please you does in fact please you and I hope I have that desire in all that I am doing.
I hope that I will never do anything apart from that desire and I know that if I do this you will lead me by the right road though I may know nothing about it.

Therefore, I will trust you always. Though I may seem to be lost and in the shadow of death, I will not fear, for you are ever with me, and will never leave me to face my perils alone.

- The Blessing of Aaron:

The Lord bless you and keep you; The Lord make his face shine upon you, and be gracious to you; the Lord lift up his countenance on you, and give you peace (Numbers 6:22–27).

Jewish Prayer

- Likely inappropriate for a non-Jewish nurse to offer. A prayer can be read from Hebrew Scripture (see the following).

* * *

Jewish (Hebrew Scripture) or Christian (Old Testament) Readings

- Psalms are poetic prayers that name the facets of the human condition and then submit the believer to Providence. Any Psalm that describes God's goodness, guidance, and protection can comfort (e.g., Psalms 18:1–24; 23; 34; 46:1–3; 63; 90; 91).
- Job is a book that tells the quintessential story of suffering. After Job loses all his wealth and children, he suffers from intensely painful sores that covered his body. Job has three friends who converse with him about the meaning of suffering. Glimpses into Job's psyche are inspiring, particularly Job 13:15 and 14:15–17. The story ends with God speaking out of a storm (Chapters 38–41); it prompts Job's response in Chapter 42:2–6, which reminds the reader of the sovereignty of God.
- Ecclesiastes is a book that discusses the meaning of life, often from a melancholic or sarcastic perspective. Because this is often the "space" a patient is in, it may be helpful. Chapter 3:1–8 reminds the reader that "there is a time for everything . . . including a time to be born and a time to die." The soliloquies about the meaning of life end with a conclusion in Chapter 12:12–14 to obey God.
- Isaiah 55:6–12 describes how God's ways are beyond human comprehension.
- Isaiah 40:25–31 describes the unfathomableness of the Creator and how God gives strength to the weary.
- Jeremiah 29 offers a message from God (originally to the Jews in exile) that promises God will answer prayers (verses 11–13).

Christian (New Testament) Readings

- Words of Jesus or stories about Jesus are found in the gospel books of the New Testament: Matthew, Mark, Luke, and John.

Jesus's words are in red font in "red-letter edition" Bibles. Passages comforting for the distressed and sick include:

- Matthew 7:7–12 (about how God loves to give good gifts to those who ask)
- Matthew 6:9–13 (the model "Lord's Prayer")
- Matthew 8:1–4, 5–13, and 14–17; Mark 2:1–12; Mark 5:25–34; Luke 17:11–19; John 5:1–15 (some of the short stories about Jesus's miraculous healings)
- Matthew 8:23–27 (provides another story with rich metaphor for the distressed)
- John 3:16–21 (about God's default stance being of love, not condemnation)
- John 14:1–3 (Jesus's promise to prepare a better place for believers)
- John 15:1–4, 8, or 17 (Jesus's parable of branches, urging believers to stay connected to the vine, to receive pruning, speaks to what being loved means)
- Comforting New Testament passages written by the earliest Christian missionaries (especially Paul):
  - Romans 8:18–28 and 31–39 (speak to how one's present suffering pales when considering future glory and how nothing can separate one from the love of Christ)
  - 1 Corinthians 6:19–20 (about one's body being a temple of the Holy Spirit)
  - 1 Corinthians 13 (describes what is love and reminds the reader how God is)
  - 1 Corinthians 15, especially 35–44, and the more likely heard 50–58 (describes the resurrection from the dead); see also 1 Thessalonians 5:13–18 regarding no need to grieve the dead
  - 2 Corinthians 12:7–10 (a role modeling of how to relate to or interpret suffering—"when I am weak, then I am strong")
  - Ephesians 2:4–10 (the classic passage describing how it is through grace by faith that the believer is saved)
  - Philippians 4:4–7 (often quoted passage about praying one's anxiety away)
  - Hebrews 11 (a long chapter listing examples of faith-filled role models who died, reminding the reader in the final two verses of how their reward is yet to come)
  - Hebrews 12:1–11 (encouragement and understanding for those who suffer)
  - James 1:2–3 (reminder to frame trials as testing and be joyful for them)
  - James 5:13–16 (admonishes to pray when in trouble; passage provides basis for anointing)

Index

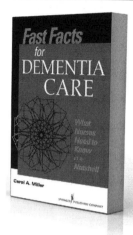
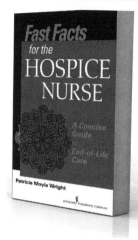
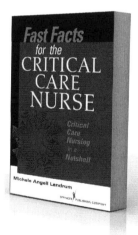
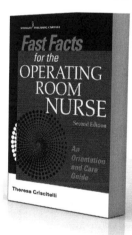